HOW TO WATCH PORN, HAVE ANAL SEX AND CALL HER BEST FRIEND FOR A THREESOME

WHAT IT TAKES TO BUILD A TRUSTING (AND FUN!) SEXUAL RELATIONSHIP

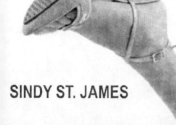

SINDY ST. JAMES

HOW TO GET HER TO WATCH PORN, HAVE ANAL SEX, AND CALL HER BEST FRIEND FOR A THREESOME

WHAT IT TAKES TO BUILD A TRUSTING (AND FUN!) SEXUAL RELATIONSHIP

by Sindy St. James

© 2008 KRE, LLC – All Rights Reserved

For more information on this series, please visit us on the web at
SecretLifePublishing.com

ISBN 978-0-9818039-5-1

KRE, LLC
PO Box 121135
Nashville, TN 37212-1135

CONTENTS

Introduction 1

Chapter 1: What Lies Beneath: Her Fears 5

Chapter 2: Your Approach: What To Say and How to Say It 18

Chapter 3: A Word About Her Excitement Levels..................................33

Chapter 4: Helping Her Ease Into Exploring New Frontiers..................35

Chapter 5: Exploring A Whole New World: Role Playing 42

Chapter 6: Porn: Watching It and Making Your Own......................50

Chapter 7: Going Beyond Missionary 57

Chapter 8: Taking It Up a Notch 79

Chapter 9: Exploring the Fringe of All Things Kinky 94

Chapter 10: Inviting Others to Play 102

Conclusion 112

Introduction

Since the dawn of time, nothing on earth has proven to be more mysterious to mankind than women. From Eve to Cleopatra to Jezebel to Britney Spears, men have never known why women do what they do or how they're going to react. Just when you think you've got it all figured out, along comes one more pretty young thing to prove you wrong – and it's back to the drawing board.

It's enough to drive you crazy!

And nowhere are women more unfathomable than in the bedroom. With guys, it's easy – guys just plain love sex, and usually don't need to be told twice to hit the sack. But girls are like a Rubik's cube – you try a million different combinations, and then all of a sudden you find you've unlocked the code and won. You have no idea how you did it, and you'd be hard pressed to do it again the same way. You know that even if you were handed the cube again with the same starting point, you'd never be able to replicate your success.

Even if you're in a relationship and are getting sex regularly, taking it to the next level can be a minefield of insecurity, arguments and outright denial of the nookie. Couples who are in perfect agreement about every aspect of their relationship can hit a dead end in the bedroom.

HOW TO GET HER TO...

Well, guys, I'll let you in on a little secret about women and sex – unless you suddenly appear from the bathroom dressed like The Gimp, your girlfriend's reticence to experiment in bed is usually NOT your fault. Simply put, women basically approach sex in a different way.

You could follow top ten lists and sure-fire tips, tricks and secrets until the cows come home – but, unless you understand where women are coming from when it comes to sex, nothing on earth is going to make them do what you want to do in bed.

And that's what this book is about – understanding what's behind that resistance, so that you can make her feel comfortable enough with you to try some new things during your next roll in the hay.

• • •

First, let's take a look at the different kinds of women out there. From my research and experience, they fall into a few categories, sexually speaking:

- **The Late Bloomer.** She might be inexperienced, she might have been hurt badly before, or she might be just plain shy. You find yourself taking it really slowly with her.

- **The Normal Girl.** She's a sexually healthy female, but she's not really into anything too crazy and likes a bit of romance in the mix. You're never really sure whether she's into sex, or just wants to please you.

- **The Tantalizer.** She kisses her girlfriends at bars and tends to kick it up a notch when she's had a few drinks; but when it comes down to the nitty gritty she'll probably find a reason not to get too crazy.

- **The Wild Child.** She might not give you much indication while out and about, but get her into a bedroom and she's ready to rock. She's got sexual confidence to spare, and she's up for almost anything. Almost.

I'm sure you've known your fair share of these women, and they can be as different as night and day. But would it surprise you to learn than deep down, they have much more in common than you'd think?

It's true. As a woman, I'm loathe to lump us all in one big basket – but really, it's just a matter of degrees when it comes to your partner's level of sexual confidence. We're all starting from the same basic insecurities, and at some point we learn how to deal with them – with varying success.

It's why you can see a tall girl who struts her stuff like a supermodel, and another one who slouches and seems embarrassed to be as tall as the guys.

It's why you can see an overweight girl who tries to hide beneath baggy clothing and wants to disappear in a corner, and another one who's showing off her cleavage and proud of the junk in her trunk.

It's why you're surprised when you realize that the girl you've been talking to barely comes up to your chest, while her friend of equally short stature seemed like a tiny mouse from the moment you met.

It's all a matter of comfort, fear and perceived limitations. Once you can see it for what it is, you're on your way to understanding women.

Chapter 1: What Lies Beneath: Her Fears

Different types, different comfort levels, but common fears and limitations – what's a boy to do when he wants to ease his ladylove into sexual encounters of the experimental kind?

Let's get into these common fears. They might not manifest in the same way from woman to woman, but chances are you've seen these in action at some point, even if you weren't able to put your finger on it – no, I don't mean that literally.

Body Image

Oh God, are we really starting with this one? Yes, Junior. It's been talked about to death in the media, but it's as real, and as common, as you'd feared – and it's the number one thing that keeps women from being less inhibited in bed.

Women are self-conscious enough with their clothes on. Chances are, by the time you meet up with your girl for date night, she's looked at herself in half a dozen outfits from every conceivable angle, and has tweezed, shaved, plucked, moisturized, perfumed or otherwise tended to every inch of her body. Then, just for kicks, she's checked out her reflection in every shiny surface from her house to yours. It's not vanity; it's sheer terror driving a woman to do things in the name of beauty that would send even the strongest man running for the hills.

So, after all this, she's got to get undressed – which, contrary to all you hold dear, is the worst moment of her evening.

That's right! For the most part, women don't realize that once the circumstances dictate that the clothes are to come off, she's already won. I mean, let's be honest here, especially among those of you with steady Betties – how often in your sexually active life have you gotten a girl to come to bed with you, and then been completely NOT into sex once she's taken off her clothes and slid in next to you?

For girls, it's the opposite. They think that once you see them up close and personal, every flaw they've managed to hide with smoke and mirrors will be magnified times a hundred.

I know it makes no sense. But that is the way female body image works.

And really, can you blame them? I don't want to get into a huge argument here about how every single aspect of a girl's environment, from the time she can walk and talk, places the value of beauty above all else, or else we'll be here until next Sunday. But, let's put it this way, as simply as possible: Men can be sexy and desirable while showing considerably less skin, and being considerably less perfectly formed, than women.

The Slut Factor

Oh man, is this fear like a loaded weapon or what? But again, it's very real, and the reasoning for it is complicated,

What Lies Beneath: Her Fears

so put on your thinking cap – you know, the one with the beer holders and two straws – and pay attention.

Some girls are sluts. We've seen slutty behavior in girls from early on – the girls who sold kisses to boys for 5 cents in grade school, for example – and we see it today, from the bar bathroom at closing time to spring break antics caught on film.

Most girls, however, are not sluts. More importantly, they never, ever, EVER want to be labeled as a slut (much to your discontent, I'm sure). And do you know why?

Because non-sluts have heard how you guys talk about sluts. Non-sluts have talked among themselves about sluts in a similar way, and none of it is particularly complimentary to the sluts in question.

Moreover, and again, not to get all anthropological on you, society has clearly spoken regarding the fate of sluts:

- Sluts become strippers in seedy bars.
- Sluts become hookers in the bad part of town.
- Sluts get raped, and no one believes them because they're sluts.
- Sluts get pregnant, and have abortions.
- Sluts wind up with The Wrong Guy.
- Sluts can't be trusted.

Given all that, non-sluts really have no interest in doing anything that might be deemed even remotely slut-like.

You might think that the cliché "lady in the living room, tiger in the bedroom" would be apt here, and would absolve a non-slut of her sins. Many women would love to have that dichotomy in a relationship, but years of social conditioning does not a cliché break.

Simply put, they think you're not going to respect them in the morning if they slut out at night.

Fear of Rejection
This one is tricky, especially for couples that have been together for a while – when you've seen someone through even the worst or most awkward of times, it'd be hard to believe that there would be a chance of rejection. But, it's something women worry about.

To a certain extent, the slut factor comes into play here. They're terrified that the life they're building with you will come crashing down once you've seen them doing something they consider taboo.

Body image fears are present here as well – they're really not sure how they would look dressed in latex with a ball gag in their mouth, but they're not going to find out while you're standing there looking at them.

Also, a girl just plain doesn't want to get laughed at in bed.

Believe it or not, her biggest fear of rejection is directly related to your penis. Sure, women have physical indicators of their level of excitement, but nothing quite stands up and says HI, I'M EXCITED, better than a penis. They'll say a lot of things to the contrary, but when it comes down to it, knowing how to make a guy sexually excited, and seeing that physical proof, is a big power trip for women.

So their fear is that, in trying something that's new and strange, they're not sure how YOU will react – and if Mister Poppy doesn't show his happy face, they will have failed in some way.

I told you, it's tricky.

Emotional Attachment
This one isn't a fear, per se, but it is something that makes a woman decline the naughtier bits of an evening's fun.

The level of emotional attachment a women needs to feel in order to be comfortable and feel confident in bed varies wildly – not only from woman to woman, but from time to time with any given partner. That being said, I'm going to go ahead and state for the record that the cliché is true:

All women, to some extent, relate sexual success to emotional investment.

Of course, getting a woman to actually admit that could result in physical harm to your manhood. But, at some level, for each and every one of us, it really is true.

Women value the physical, emotional and spiritual connection during the sexual act. And many things that are experimental in nature require that connection to be broken – to varying degrees and for varying lengths of time, but still broken.

So, that's not going to be high on their list of bedroom to-dos.

• • •

There are more specific, and more serious, reasons why certain women are not going to be into bedroom escapades. Let's go over them now, just to get them out there.

Past Sexual Abuse
I'm really not sure what on God's green earth is more devastating than a wonderful, giving, loving woman with a history of sexual abuse. Whether it was from within the family, a trusted adult, a later relationship with a boyfriend or husband, or a rape or date rape experience, a woman who has been sexually abused needs all the strength she can muster to lead any semblance of a normal life.

So, while many sexually abused women do go on to lead healthy sex lives, it is absolutely imperative that there are open lines of communication between you regarding any sexual act.

Body Image, Part Two
I know, I know. You thought we were done in the last section. But there is another whole level of body issues that you should be aware of that goes beyond the whole "does my ass look fat in this" vibe girls seem to love inflicting on their men.

Sometimes – and frankly, more often than you realize – women can take their insecurities about their body image to a dangerous place.

Anorexia is an example of this. An anorexic woman is not going to want you to see her naked, for two very mixed-up reasons: one, she thinks you're going to tell her she's too fat; two, she thinks you are going to tell her she's too thin. Yes, I know they're the opposite. But that's just the tip of the iceberg with this debilitating disease.

Bulimia is another example. That's where a woman will eat normal meals with others, or binge in private, and then throw it all up as soon as possible (before the food has time to digest). A bulimic woman's mindset is similar to the anorexic's in that she's going to be worried you'll think she's fat. But, there are reasons specific to bulimia that will make her keep her pants on.

First off, if you're bringing home a woman with bulimia after a dinner date and expecting to take her to bed, it's not going to happen. She either didn't have time to purge, in which case she's feeling way too fat to see herself naked, let alone you see her; or she did purge while you weren't noticing, and probably feels badly about it and just wants to be alone.

Also, chronic bulimia tends to cause halitosis, and can bloat the stomach – two things that will keep a bulimic woman self-conscious enough to stay away from your firm embrace.

Body Image, Part Three
I know this whole section is such a downer, but it's important to be aware of the stuff going on behind the veneer – and I promise this is the last body image thing I'll talk about so seriously.

Have you ever heard of cutting? It's where a girl will purposely cut herself – not to kill herself, but tiny ritualistic cuts in different parts of her body, usually places that can be easily hidden by clothing. If you've ever seen the movie Secretary, I'm talking about what Maggie Gyllenhall's character did to herself.

The reasons why girls cut themselves in this horrific manner are not always directly related to body image. I'm sure I don't have to tell you that, even if a woman has been treated for cutting and no longer does it, it's going to leave scars – emotional and physical – that she will be extremely reticent about letting you see.

Conflicting Religious Beliefs
Yeah, yeah, I know – Catholic schoolgirls blah, blah, blah. Take it from one of them – those nuns do a number on your psyche. I once had a nun give me a pretty solid argument for why chewing gum leads to pregnancy!

All joking aside, though, strictly held religious beliefs really aren't up for debate, especially if those beliefs have to do with sexual conduct.

If the woman you're with has been brought up in a devoutly religious environment, she's going to bring a lot of baggage to any discussion about sexual experimentation. And, if she is still devout as an adult, you're going to come up against even more resistance.

You're going to need to tread lightly – very lightly. You don't want to be seen as Satan's minion. And you really don't want to offend what is a very real relationship she has with her faith.

Bad Men

Many women have had crappy relationships with men who were really, really wrong for them. They are not the bad men I'm talking about here. The bad men I'm talking about now are mean. They might have sexually, physically, and/or emotionally abused a woman during their relationship.

If your girlfriend or wife has been in an abusive relationship in her adult life, chances are you'll know it. It's not going to be the usual bitching about what an asshole he was – she might flinch at your sudden movement, or automatically go into a defensive stance when you were just going in for a hug. She might have a serious freak out if you come home sauced from a night with the guys and want some nookie. Or, maybe she will be terrified when she breaks something or when you raise your voice to her.

You have to do everything you can to let her know that she can trust you, and that you trust her.

If you are with a woman who has had any experiences like the ones described in this section, the advice in this book will be helpful to you – but for the most part, we're going to be talking about otherwise sexually healthy women.

For these women above, though, you'd be wise to let a lot – and I mean, A LOT – of very quiet, very understanding, very trusting conversations happen before you even contemplate broaching the subject of sexual experimentation. Conversations in which you gently ask questions, and then shut up and listen – no typical "I'll solve this problem" man-thinking here.

• • •

The thing is, guys, we love you. You're our boyfriends and husbands. We are crazy about you. We want to be that tiger in the bedroom if it drives you wild with passion, and we want to be the only one you come running to when you need to scratch that kinky itch.

So, depending on the type of woman you've got between the sheets, you're going to get different signals that will let you know that no, she really is not interested in the hot wax treatment on her nipples. Let's go back to our four basic types:

You're going to get the most physical resistance from the **Late Bloomer**. She'll freeze up, and become really tense. She might stop talking or kissing you. She might leave the bed, or suggest doing something else entirely that has nothing to do with sex.

The **Normal Girl** is going to be a bit nervous, and might treat your suggestions like a joke and laugh them off, then gently steer you back toward whatever more traditional thing you two were doing. She's not going to want to talk about it too much afterward, either.

The **Tantalizer** will deflect your experimental nature by proposing something else that she feels more comfortable with – a strip tease, maybe, or some particular trick she knows you love. She's going to be more open to talking about your desires than most girls, at least, even if it's all talk – because she is smart enough to know that just talking about it, and wondering if she'll go along with it, is going to turn you on.

The **Wild Child** is probably going to be game for some pretty far-out stuff. If she's not into what you want to do, she'll tell you – and give you her reasons. However, the Wild Child probably has some kinks of her own – which is a great starting point in communication that we'll get into a bit later in the book.

Of course, with any of our girls here, she might just surprise you and go along with it right off the bat – but you've got to be aware of their comfort level.

- Did she go along with it, but just isn't into it?
- Does she seem bored?
- Is she trying to hurry you to orgasm?
- Is she making fake porn star sounds?
- Does she rush out of bed immediately afterward?
- How open is she to talking about it afterward?

These are just a few of the things for which you should be looking. But, you know her better than I do – so be on the lookout for any sign that she's not comfortable, and hold off on the kinks for now.

• • •

Oops, another word here before we get into the heart of the matter:

Sexual experimentation can be a wonderful component of any solid relationship. A little kink now and then can spice up your sex life. Especially after a couple has been together a while, when sex can seem less like the shiny new toy that it was when you first met.

The advice in this book is aimed at loving couples in long-term relationships. We're not talking about plain old sex here – we're talking about easing your partner into trying new things that are a little more extreme than what the two of you are used to doing in the bedroom (or kitchen, or car, or beach…).

In other words, there are three situations in which the advice and suggestions in this book should NOT be used:

1. One-night stands or very new, very casual relationships. We're going to be talking a lot about trust, communication and several levels of experimentation over a long period of time. There is no speed course here. If you try to take a shortcut with a fling to get your kink on, you're going to wind up in trouble.

2. Long-term relationships that are in crisis or have deep-seated problems. Success in sexual experimentation depends on a rock-solid foundation of trust and mutual respect. If you and your woman have issues, I can't stress how important it is that you work them out – not only for our purposes, but for the good of your relationship in the long term.

O.K. As Marvin Gaye once said: Let's get it on.

Chapter 2: Your Approach: What To Say and How to Say It

They might show it in wildly different ways, but at their core, women are nurturers. They speak in terms of safe havens, comfort zones, closure, release, nesting, fulfillment, and a variety of other phrases that make you think of hot cocoa and snuggling under blankets.

Which is why you have no idea what they're talking about half of the time.

And that's O.K. If they were just like you, you probably wouldn't be half as interested in them as you are!

But, if you've got a special lady in your life and you'd like to take your bedroom activities to the next level, it's extremely important that you really, really understand the female mindset.

We've already talked about general types of women, and some of the major reasons why they're reluctant to become Little Miss Nasty for you. Now, we're going to do something about it!

Keeping in mind what kind of woman you're with – **The Late Bloomer, The Normal Girl, The Tantalizer** or **The Wild Child** – your first step is to start talking about sex.

This will also be your second step, your third step, and your 400th step. You're going to have to rinse and repeat until your girl feels comfortable enough to let loose in bed.

A lot of guys hope they can kind of slide in a kinky thing or two while they're having sex, but that's the worst possible time to do it. If you're serious about wanting to include your partner in some experimenting, you're going to have to do it the hard way – no pun intended.

Before I get into when you should broach the subject of sexual experimentation, I'd like to give you a list of when NOT to talk about it. Many instances on this list will make absolutely no sense to you, but I'll walk you through it.

You should note that there are obvious exceptions to these, and it's always best to trust the parameters of your relationship. I'm giving worst-case scenarios here, and their overarching theme is that women, in their nurturing ways, are inclined to obsess, worry and analyze, because they are very, very attentive to their men and those around them.

That's because their nurturing ways want to please you. And, in their minds, if you want to do something other than whatever you're already doing in the bedroom, they're not pleasing you. It's as simple as that.

So, these times below are when you run the risk of her thinking that you are less than happy with your sex life.

HOW TO GET HER TO...

DO NOT TALK ABOUT SEX OR SEXUAL EXPERIMENTATION FOR THE FIRST TIME:

When other people are present. She'll be pissed at you for embarrassing her. Then, every time you bring it up after that, she'll only remember that one time you embarrassed her.

After you've been at any gathering together at which some seriously hot women were present. She's going to think you would rather be tying that model to the bed.

When either of you have been drinking or are drunk. It'll be written off as the blathering of a drunken idiot and you'll never be taken seriously. Or, she'll think you got her drunk to take advantage of her. Yes, this holds true even if you've been together for a long time.

On the way home after having been out with other people, in particular another couple, especially if the subject of sexual experimentation was discussed at any time during the evening. She's going to think you compared your relationship to someone else's, found yours lacking, and want to experiment because you're bored. Or, that you're fantasizing about one of the women present, and want to do whatever she was talking about to your girlfriend and pretend it's that other woman.

After you have come home from a boys' night out. See "not while you're drunk" above. Also, she'll think you're trying to one-up your mates by doing something you all giggled about like schoolboys, and then bring them back salacious tales of her sluttiness.

Immediately before having sex. This will have her wondering in panic the whole time if you'd rather be doing something, or someone, else.

During sex. She's in the zone. Don't mess with her. She'll think she's not doing it right or that you can't get it up and are making excuses.

Immediately after having sex. She'll think you didn't enjoy it and will make her less inclined to have sex with you again anytime soon for fear of not pleasing you.

During or immediately after watching a television show or film that talks about or portrays sexual experimentation. You might think this is a good time, but only if SHE brings it up first as being really hot. Girls look at hot scenes on TV and in movies differently than guys do; girls are wondering how often the girl works out, or if she was embarrassed to have to disrobe in front of the crew, or how many takes they did of the scene. Guys are thinking, OMG BOOBIES.

When she's caught you looking at porn and/or masturbating. Duh.

When she's caught you cheating on her. Double duh.

Before, during or after any serious talk about the future of your relationship. This will make her think that any terms, negotiations or moving ahead you're doing is contingent on her bringing the nasty to the bedroom.

HOW TO GET HER TO...

Before, during or after either of your relatives visit, especially parents. There is simply way too much baggage that comes with relatives. She's going to be in full perfect child, hostess or girlfriend mode, which is not a sexy frame of mind. (However, if you are the kind of couple who get off while getting it on in your parents' bedroom, then this would be the perfect time.)

Before or after any vacation you take together, or that you take without her. Before a vacation together, she's going to worry the whole time that you want her to do whatever it is you talked about, and that you're not having a good time. After, she'll think you didn't have a good time. On one without her – well, she really doesn't want to hear anything except how much you will/did miss her.

Before, during or after any relationship anniversary she acknowledges, no matter how meaningless to you. This includes Christmas, her birthday, and Valentine's Day (no matter what she says). Women take anniversaries and holidays very seriously. She's already going to be worried that you're not as much into the holiday as she is, and anything you say about sexual experimentation is going to come out of left field for her.

Anniversaries and Valentine's Day is about romance and gifts. She must be the sole focus of her birthday, and there must be gifts. Christmas – gifts. If sex is in any way suggested as a gift, she will think you are being cheap. Any sex must be in addition to gifts, and romantic in nature.

And Thanksgiving. She's going to be feeling fat and there will probably be relatives involved. And she's going to be bitter about doing all the work that goes into entertaining (yes, even if you're guests at someone else's dinner). Anything involving sex will seem like another chore. The only exception to this is if you whisk her off on a vacation over the long weekend.

And Mardi Gras. News stories about drunk girls flashing their tits for beads is not going to get her in the mood. Shocking, I know.

And New Year's Eve. See "not while you're drunk" above. She wants you to keep her Champagne glass full and kiss her at midnight. That's about all she can handle on a night as emotional as New Year's. Women tend to recall all the times they didn't have anyone to kiss, and they want the night to be about romance.

From a few days before to a few days after any wedding you attend together. She'll think you're panicking about a lifetime of sex with the same woman, and trying to feel like you're still a wild and crazy guy.

At any time starting from the moment you are engaged until you die. O.K., this one is an exaggeration. But seriously, any kinks in the relationship – pun absolutely intended – should be worked out BEFORE you pop the question. Anything after that point will be seen as panicking (see above), and disregarded.

Or, you might freak her out: "How could he have hidden this from me? What else is he hiding from me? Am I really going to agree to spend the rest of my life with someone who hides sick shit like this from me until the last second? Do I even know him?"

Or, you'll overwhelm and annoy her: "I've got final fittings for my dress, my florist bailed and now he wants me to dress like a French maid and step on his back in stilettos? Give me a break, I don't have time for this."

When she is sick, doing household chores, running errands, or any other time she is not looking and feeling her best. The last thing she is thinking about is having sex, let alone trying something new and inventive. She's going to see it like one more thing she has to do for you.

O.K., so that was a lot to take in. Go ahead and read them again, this time without shaking your head in disbelief.

Now we get to move onto the good part: finally getting up the courage to talk to her about what you desire most in the bedroom.

Remember how I said that women's nurturing ways mean they want to please you? I do mean that, but not in the honey-get-me-a-sandwich kind of way. They want to know that they complete you, fulfill you, and are the only one in your life.

So, the times to bring up the down and dirty stuff are during or, even better, after you have reminded her that she is your end all and be all.

APPROPRIATE TIMES TO BRING UP SEX AND SEXUAL EXPERIMENTATION FOR THE FIRST TIME:

A day or so after you've had really great sex. (With her.) It's important to make sure she knows how awesome the sex was immediately afterward. Make sure your praise evolves into how great you feel about the relationship. Then, go into how you feel close enough with her to reveal your kinky side.

On vacation. (With her, and only her.) This works best if you're on a particularly luxurious vacation or somewhere exotic; less so if you're backpacking through the Alps in a rainstorm. But, either way, a vacation is an ideal opportunity to bring up your naughty ideas. You're out of your own element, so you're not going to be interrupted or distracted by life's little moments. You're hopefully having a lot of great, relaxed sex during which you're really connecting. And you're spending more time with each other, which thrills her and enables you to be able to read her better for the perfect moment to talk about whatever it is you're interested in trying.

First thing in the morning, particularly on a weekend. Now, I know that some women can be absolute beasts in the morning – I'm one of them. But there's something about being able to wake up next to your love on a lazy Saturday or Sunday, and whiling away an hour or so talking about whatever pops into your head. Also, an excellent time to recount sex dreams involving her as a segue. You want to make sure you tell her that you've never thought about it before, but it really made you hot, and how weird it was.

While you're at a video store. It can be done as a dare, as partners in crime, or just as a joke – but getting her into the porn section of a video store is actually a pretty good way to talk about sex. You can kid around about the awful titles, be scandalized by the really raunchy stuff, and then find something that actually does turn you on. Don't pressure her into renting anything – but the trip home from the store, you can bring it up again. "No, seriously though, that one video…"

Walking by a shop that sells sex toys. Not a porn store, but one of those fun and flirty sex toy shops that cater to women and parties. When you're waking by during a particularly easygoing day, drag her in – then follow the examples given above for the video store.

A minimum of four days after: a wedding you attend, visiting relatives leave, important-to-her holidays, anytime you're both out and someone else brings it up, a party attended by hot women, vacations, etc. Waiting so long gives you two advantages: one, she won't connect your bringing it up with whatever the event was; two, if she does connect it, you can appear to have really thought about it in the context of your relationship as opposed to a knee-jerk reaction to something.

Before Halloween. Go looking for costumes together. Follow the examples for the video and sex toy stores above.

After she's gone to a naughty bachelorette party. This works if your kink or fetish is cuckolding, and the party featured a male stripper. It also works only if your lady was into it.

Or sex toy party. (Think R-rated Tupperware party). Usually a sexpert is brought in to help sell sex toys at an informal cocktail gathering of women. If she comes home having responded positively to the frank sex talk she's heard, she'll never be more ready to hear what you've got to say.

• • •

There are more examples on both ends of the spectrum, of course, but I just wanted to give you an idea of the sense of timing with which you need to handle the broaching of such a delicate subject.

Now that you've got an idea of the right moment to talk to her, let's cover what you're going to say – and more importantly, how you're going to say it.

Again, like waiting for the right time, much of your choice is going to depend on the general kind of woman you're with and the particular circumstances of your relationship.

It also depends on what kind of sexual experimentation you're looking to engage in with her. But, we'll get into those specifics in a bit. For right now, we're going back to the psychology of communicating with your ladylove about loving your lady.

Story time!

I grew up in a pretty straitlaced environment, and didn't start having sex until I got to college when, for the better part of those four years – and even for a few years after – I had a steamy affair with a film major whom we'll call Leo.

Leo and I connected on many levels, and we're still very close friends today. But pretty much everything we both know about sex, experimental and otherwise, we learned together – in our dorm rooms, on staircases, in editing suites, on bathroom sinks… you get the idea.

One day, when no one else was around, he said he had something he wanted to ask me, and he would be 100 percent O.K. with my answer no matter what I said.

His filmmaking professor assigned a free-form project that could be on any topic. He said he was thinking about submitting a porn film – and that there was no one on earth he trusted more than me to make it with him. He then went on to explain his concept, which was a funny story about two people of varying heights trying to have sex standing up. It would be shot in one take and be just a few minutes long, I'd be shot from the shoulders down, and he would let me see it before he showed it to the class. If I was in any way uncomfortable with the final product he would take the pass.

I said yes immediately, despite my absolute terror at doing something that five minutes before would never have crossed my mind. And do you know why?

Because he explicitly said that he trusted me. He said there was no one on earth he trusted more, in fact.

Now, I'm not saying that the rest of what he said didn't

appeal to me – the screening, my face not being shown. And, of course it helped that I trusted him too, and knew he was an otherwise upstanding guy.

But the words that sealed the deal were, "There is no one on earth I trust more than you."

This delightful tale of college-age debauchery is to illustrate my point that the foundation of any sexual experimentation must be trust. It is the single most important feeling to instill in your partner, and it must be explicit, not implicit.

• • •

Do something for me right now – think about a time when you and your wife or girlfriend had great sex. Replay it in your mind for a few seconds. (I know, I ask you to do the most difficult things.)

What do you remember about it? Her body, the sounds she made, maybe the moment in which you had an orgasm?

Women think of the physical aspects of sex, too, but with those memories come intense feelings of the emotional or even spiritual connection she experienced. Those feelings need to be present in order for a woman to not only have a positive sexual experience, but to continue to think of that experience in a positive way.

No matter how great the sex is for her on an immediate, visceral level, whatever happens both before and after it is

HOW TO GET HER TO...

also taken into account as she decides whether or not it was a positive experience in the long run.

Trusting you is an integral part of that experience. I sincerely hope your relationship is based on mutual trust and respect. But, sexual experimentation takes that understanding to a different level. And, if done correctly, in many ways it can confirm and even build on that trust.

All of this has to come through in every conversation you have with your partner about sexual experimentation.

However, the key is to always be yourself. That conversation I had with Leo was a serious one – he wasn't joking around, flirting with me or tricking me – but he was still the same Leo, and his sincerity was obvious. He understood the importance of what he was asking me to do and at the same time had no shame about it whatsoever. Even now, on the rare occasions we remember it or joke about it, he always talks about it with respect and admiration.

But I'm guessing you're not a film student with an upcoming porn project, so enough about Leo – let's get back to you.

・・・

While I will never recommend trickery when trying to get your woman to experiment in bed, there will be some clever conversational tactics you can employ to get her to play along with your reindeer games.

Your Approach: What To Say and How to Say It

Here are some things to keep in mind:

- Always keep the focus on the two of you doing it together, as true partners in sex.

- No matter what your prior experience is, NEVER, UNDER ANY CIRCUMSTANCES, can you tell her about other girlfriends who've been into being dirty with you. Never. EVER. Lie, if you have to, within reason.

- Keep calm when you're talking about it, especially after she becomes more open to the idea. You don't want to act like a kid who just got a puppy.

- The same goes for including her in the conversation – keep her involved, and LISTEN to her. Don't just ask her a question so that she'll ask you back, and give you your chance to unload everything.

- Be open and understanding to what she's saying – no judgments, no laughing AT her, no being embarrassed. She might tell you things that she's ashamed of, or that she has been told are bad or weird. Reward her trust in you.

Depending on what your kink is, you're going to want to start slowly, and then ease off – both when talking the talk and walking the walk. Let each conversation take its own direction, and don't push the issue. If she's clearly uncomfortable, let it drop and wait a while to bring it up again in a different way later.

And for goodness sake, lighten it up! Everyone has sex, and things that seem perfectly normal to one couple might seem weird or extreme to another. The perfect timing, and the perfect words, should come as easy to you as talking about the party you're going to or the errands you have to run together this weekend.

Above all else, remember that for now, you're just talking here. You're not going to have a four-minute conversation and then progress immediately to swinging from the chandelier while being tickled with a feather. It just doesn't work that way – not if you want it to become a regular part of your sexual repertoire!

Besides, the more she opens up to the idea, the hotter the talking part will become!

CHAPTER 3: A Word About Her Excitement Levels

It might not seem like it right now, but once you finish learning about how to bring your partner into the world of sexual experimentation, you might find that you've created your own Wild Child!

There are a few things that can happen when a woman is having sex, and I'd like to mention them here as a way to emphasize the role communication plays in even the hottest of moments.

- Queefing – When you're thrusting in and out of her vagina, the change in air pressure and suction will cause it to emit a fart-like sound. It can be seriously embarrassing for her, and it might make you laugh. Tell her your penis did that to her, and move on.

- Farting – Kind of like queefs during anal sex, or sometimes it can be just a bit of gas while you're concentrating on other areas of her body. Again, embarrassing – and maybe smelly! Tell her it's normal and drop the subject forever – this means no referring to it later, even in veiled references.

- Female ejaculation – You might be fascinated by it, and depending on your skills you might even be able to facilitate it (by applying movement and pressure to the ridged area about halfway into her vagina). But whether it's the first time it happens or it happens all the time, it's one of the most embarrassing things for girls EVER. That's because a lot of liquid tends to come out, and a less knowledgeable person might think she's peed herself.

If your girl female ejaculates – first of all, nice one! It usually only happens when girls are super excited! But secondly, and more importantly, please let her know that you know that she hasn't peed herself, and that you don't mind all the liquid everywhere. Play it way cool, hold her afterward and kiss her, and don't make fun of her for it – EVER.

Chapter 4: Helping Her Ease Into Exploring New Frontiers

I keep harping on about talking and taking it slowly, because guys tend to go right for the thing they want the second they get even an inkling of a green light from their woman. It's all about baby steps, and working up to the stuff that really floats your boat.

Let's jump right into it with an example a common fetish – like having sex in public. There's a bit of thrill to it, it involves both partners equally, and there is no apparatus needed (usually!). And, the worst that can happen? You'll get caught, and maybe given a ticket by a cop for indecent exposure. No one's going to get hurt.

Let's walk through the process of getting your woman on board with a nice shag in the great outdoors.

First, think about any particular needs she has for your run-of-the-mill sexual activity.

- Does she always make you turn off the lights?

- Does she get nervous if she hears voices or car doors slamming nearby?

- Does she keep pretty quiet during sex, and get embarrassed if you get a bit noisy?

- Does she tell you to slow down if the headboard starts banging?

- If someone interrupts (phone call, visitor, etc.), is she mortified? Does she make you swear you won't say what you two have been doing?

These are all signs that she's probably not ready for the world at large to acknowledge you're having sex, WHILE you're having sex. So, saying flat-out that you want to ravage her in the men's room during a concert is really not going to get her juices flowing. She'll flat-out tell you you're crazy!

Getting your ladylove to go along with your sexual experimentation is a lot like dating and then getting serious with her. It's all about the wooing at first, but you want to keep that spark alive, even when you've moved in together and you've seen each other every single day for a year. Do you get what I mean? You don't want to go too far, too fast.

However, it is good to acknowledge that you have this fetish, and that your fantasy is to one day do it with her. Tell her why you get so turned on by it – maybe it's because you think you guys are so hot together, you want the world to know! Or, maybe it is the risk factor, or the urgency needed. Maybe you get turned on at concerts, and dream of "doing it" while your favorite song is being played live!

Helping Her Ease Into Exploring New Frontiers

Then, ask her what her fantasies are. If she says she doesn't have any, ask again – but if she gets really embarrassed or nervous, gently let it go.

During your next few sessions of lovemaking, raise the bar a bit.

If she likes it pitch black, maybe light some candles, then advance to having a nice lamp on while having sex. Tell her how beautiful she is, and that you want to see her while you're making love to her. Afterward, make sure she knows how much it meant to you that she let you do that – it really meant a lot.

If you live alone, or if you know your housemates will absolutely NOT be back for a long time, try having sex with your bedroom door open, then have sex in the shower or bath, move gradually to the kitchen counter, maybe, or the sofa. (Not all in one night, stud – over the course of several weeks! Take it slow.) Make sure she knows that no one will be back for a while, and make sure she trusts you on that one. Again, the element of trust is big here.

Once she is perfectly comfortable having sex in the house this way, then you can start to take it outside. Again, this is to be done slowly, gradually, over some time. Choose times and places that make her comfortable, and get in tune with her mindset at any particular time, so you're hitting the right marks with her. And, as always, make her feel safe – that by doing this with you, she has no reason to fear or be embarrassed.

HOW TO GET HER TO...

Some examples of getting her comfortable with public displays of some serious affection, try some of these:

And the end of the night, have a make-out session in the car before going into the house to have sex. Make sure no one is around – you want her to be comfortable out of the safety and comfort of the bedroom and the home. But, for the first several times, always finish inside. Eventually, you can work up to having sex in the car on a private road or turn-off on the highway. Nighttime is best, when there are significantly less people around.

If she gets nervous and fidgety, and is clearly not responding, STOP. But don't be petulant about it! Just work it back down, give her a final kiss, and take her back home and ravage her. Tell her how hot it was to make out like teenagers again, and how excited it made you to see her like that. Remember, always bring it back to her and making her feel good about what you two have done.

At parties, take her aside for a moment for a steamy kiss. Let her know from your actions that you're not going to do anything that makes her feel uncomfortable – you just wanted to sneak in a quick kiss, maybe a little feel. When you go back to the crowd, hold her hand and be gentle with her, pay attention to her – or, at the very least, if you get separated, give her a few steamy looks from across the room. Make her feel wanted, and make sure she knows that what you two did pleased you greatly.

A day in the park or the beach can also escalate the stakes, once you're sure she's absolutely OK with everything you've done so far. Go for a swim together, and kiss her in the water. Duck behind a tree for a quick kiss (nothing more, at first). Spoon together on a blanket in the afternoon sun.

You're getting her comfortable with public displays. Don't act like you're sneaking around – once she sees that either no one is paying attention, or that someone who does see you simply smiles at a nice couple in love, she'll start to relax. If you do get "caught" – say, by a friend at the party who sneaks out for a smoke, or a jogger in the park – don't act urgently to stop, or be ashamed (but don't brag, either). Put your arm around her, or hold her hand, and be calm and cool about it.

"Yep, you caught us! I just can't keep my hands off this woman. She's just too beautiful." Acknowledging it will make everyone feel less awkward, and the moment will pass more quickly and be done. She'll be able to immediately see that it's no big deal.

When done gradually, with lots of times in between where you're not furthering your agenda, she will become more comfortable with the idea. Go a little further each time, slowly – first a kiss, then a lengthier kiss, then a feel here and there, then a full make-out that ends in sex in a safe place for her. Then back out, maybe a little fingering action, maybe you let her feel how hard it makes you.

Always acknowledge that it is HER that is exciting you in these situations, not THE ACT of doing it. Knowing that she pleases you so much, she'll be much more inclined to keep on taking risks with you in order to see how much she can please you.

For the time when you eventually go all the way outside in public, make sure it is as safe as possible, meaning – where there is a 100 percent chance that you WON'T get caught. As always, bring it back to her afterwards, and how excited she made you, and how close you feel to her after having done it.

If it's a place that is accessible on a regular basis, and again you're SURE you won't get caught, make it your "thing" for a while to go there and have sex. Let her feel absolutely 100 percent comfortable there.

And, of course, always intersperse these times with "plain vanilla" sex in bed, lots of whatever it is she wants to do sexually, and all the lesser things you've done along the way. Don't stop grabbing her and kissing her on the street, or sneaking her off at parties for a quick make-out. Otherwise, she'll see it all as a ruse. You've got to make her understand that all of it turns you on – that SHE turns you on, no matter what you're doing together.

Talking is always important, too – while you're making out with her at the party, whisper in her ear how turned on she makes you. Save the more dirty talk for when there is absolutely no way you will try anything with her – it will make her able to appreciate your fetish more if she knows there is no risk of you following through with it at that moment, and she can fantasize about it safely, and make it her own.

Helping Her Ease Into Exploring New Frontiers

For example, say you're taking a rest from walking at the mall. You're both sitting on the side of a fountain, or next to each other on a bench. You're holding onto some bags, or sipping on a soda.

Reach over and give her a peck on the cheek, smile at her. Tell her you love her. Let a few more minutes go by – sipping on your soda, people-watching. Then, you lean over like you're going to maybe talk about someone that just passed by, but instead you whisper to her how much you wish you could rip off her clothes, throw her in the fountain and just take her right there in front of everyone. Give her another peck, sip your soda, make a funny face at her, and then suggest it's time to keep walking.

As you and your partner become more open about sex talk, make sure to try out some of the things she wants to do as well. You've got to give as good as you get, baby!

Once again, this all comes back to trust. When she sees that you trust her enough to do whatever thing it is she wants, she's going to give it back to you in spades.

Chapter 5: Exploring A Whole New World: Role Playing

Communication and trust are also a part of the immediate sexual experience, as well. Other than what I've already mentioned – encouraging her, complimenting her, and making sure she knows that she is the one that is turning you on more than whatever it is you're doing – there are times when it's imperative that you're on the same wavelength and are communicating effectively.

Role-playing experimentation is an excellent example of the importance of communication. I'm sure you've seen funny scenes on TV and in films about using a "safe word," but for professionals and other experienced members of the fetish community, the subject of safe words is no laughing matter.

Safe words are needed any time you are doing something in which one or both partners are playing the role of someone who is reluctant – or, really, anytime conversational play or improvisation is a part of the activity. But, having a safe word even in the earlier stages of sexual experimentation can go a long way toward putting your partner at ease.

Before you start any kind of experimental play, have you and your girl agree on a safe word. It can be anything – a city name, a color, an animal, or even a phrase, like "red light." Just make sure it is not a word or phrase that can come up in context of your role playing, and don't make the word "stop."

Then, once the word is used, whatever you're doing must cease immediately. There's no negotiation on this one.

Some things to keep in mind once a safe word is used by either of you:

- First of all, don't be afraid to use it – either of you. It was invented for a reason.

- It's perfectly ok to continue to mess around and even have sex – just make sure that none of the experimental aspects are a part of it. Go back to "plain" sexual activity.

- Make her feel comfortable after the safe word has been used, no matter who used it. A simple, "OK" is fine, and lots of holding, cuddling and snuggling. A safe word is called as such because it's about safety – so you want to create a safe, comfortable zone in the time immediately following its use.

- WAIT to talk about why either she or you used it. Concentrate on recreating a safe environment, and then after all sexual activity is finished for the time being, you can talk about it.

- If she was the one that used the safe word, be absolutely understanding, patient and loving. She's going to say "I'm sorry," and this is the time you must stress that there is absolutely no need to be sorry. Work out what made her uncomfortable, and discuss how you can tone it down or change that element to make a successful time of it sometime later.

- If you were the one that used it, your actions are going to go a lot further than your words. Hold her, caress her, and make her feel loved. She's going to be vulnerable at that point, and you need to let her know that everything is O.K. Then, when you do talk about it, be calm, open and honest. If something she did freaked you out, don't lie – but make it about YOUR freak-out, not about what SHE was doing. In arriving at a solution, phrase your words so that she is the one helping you get through it, not, "You need to change this or that."

- The important thing, though, is to get back in the saddle, as they say – and when it comes to fetishes, that could be taken literally! But seriously, don't use it as an excuse to never try again. It's called sexual EXPERIMENTATION because that's just what it is – and, like all experiments, adjustments need to be made until you find the formula that works for you.

Role-playing is an interesting fetish in that, at some non-sexual level, everyone has done it before. As children we played cowboys and Indians, or "house," or dressed up in

Exploring A Whole New World: Role Playing

our parents clothes or costumes for a play. And in our lives, we play different roles, too – you're a different person with your buddies on game night than you are during an office meeting with all your bosses present.

But, many times women get turned off by role-playing. Why is that?

For one, it can lean towards the cliché – the French maid, the naughty nurse, the sexy schoolgirl or the naïve secretary are just way, way overdone. From Halloween costumes to bad porn films, women know enough about these roles to assume that your desire to see her play them is not about her, but about the costume.

So, once again, it comes down to letting her know that it is HER you want to see don the costume or play the role, not just the costume or role itself.

For another, it can be just plain embarrassing to her. Sure, in he heat of the moment, it might be sexy – but then you've finished, or you've said the safe word, and now you're two adults standing there in ridiculous costumes replaying in your head all the stupid shit you just said. That's not going to be a cherished memory for her.

That's why it is important that there be lots of soothing, encouraging activity focused on her, and without any shame in what you've just done. She needs to know that you don't think she looked or acted dumb, and that it really means a lot to you that she went along with it.

How you get your lady into role-playing really depends on the kind of role-playing you want to do. For the sake of example, let's say the extreme end of role-playing is when you set up a time in which you meet, play your roles, have sex, and leave all while in costume and in character. The stages leading up to her active and willing participation in something like that would then be the lesser versions of role-playing.

The first step is, as always, talking to her about what turns you on about role playing. See how she feels about it, and if she has ever had any similar fantasies. Maybe there was a crush on a high school teacher, or a handyman at work.

Again, make sure it stays on topic, and that it is about doing it with HER. This is especially important in role-play, as asking her to "be" another person while having sex can be misinterpreted as you being bored with her in bed.

However, if the role playing you are interested in requires her to be the dominant role – say, she's a teacher and you're a student, or you're a virgin and she's a slut or prostitute – that can be an empowering feeling for her that you would want to explore with her in conversation.

The next step is to get talking while in bed. Start with mildly dirty stuff, mostly just using explicit language at first. If you want her to say things, don't just say, "Talk dirty to me." Tell her what you want to hear: "Tell me how my big my cock is." "Tell me you're a dirty girl." Get her to repeat things after you, so she doesn't have to think much about it and get distracted from the task at hand.

Once you let her see how much that turns you on, you can get her to participate more by having her answer specific questions. "Tell me how I feel inside you." "How does it feel when I do this?" Give positive reinforcement to whatever she says, even if she's bad at it.

If she seems to be embarrassed or struggling to find words, answer it for her and have her give yes/no answers. "Can you feel my tongue here? Does it feel good?" "Do you like it when I fill you up like that?"

Make sure you move slowly on this – you don't want to be a Chatty Kathy out of nowhere. Go back to not talking during sex, and make sure to keep up the romance in between all the dirty talk. Lots of "I love you" and "You're so beautiful" should be in there, too.

If you want to get into dressing the part and costume play, go for it at Halloween with a party. Choose a theme for the both of you – or better yet, have her choose it, or go shopping for costumes together – and make it fun and flirty, but not too overtly sexual. Theme parties are good any time of the year, and can let her see that everyone loves dressing up.

Then, after the party, have sex while still wearing your costumes. Throw a little talk in there, keeping it fun and light, but don't go all out with the role-playing just yet.

Afterwards, as you're changing back into normal clothing, joke that she should keep that costume handy – you just might have to do that again sometime. Then, drop it for a while.

HOW TO GET HER TO...

Depending on what kind of role-playing you like, try to integrate it into non-sexual times in a fun and light way. If she asks you to fix something in the house, play the role of the handyman, and do some heavy flirting. Is she at the table with her glasses on, looking over some papers? Tell her she looks like a sexy librarian, and kiss her deeply. These types of things will get her used to the idea of seeing each other as characters, in safe instances where there is no pressure on her to "perform."

Conversations about role playing can be a bit like foreplay, as well, and can really get her in the mood to test the waters. If something either of you are doing reminds you of your role-playing fantasy, tell her!

"You look so sexy with your glasses on, like a sexy librarian. Come on, that's a huge fantasy of mine! I go into the library, and there you are behind your desk, all stern and buttoned up. I ask for help in the stacks, and as you reach up to grab a book for me, you stumble and I catch you…"

You get the idea. The important thing is to always make it about HER and YOU in the roles – not "a sexy librarian," but HER AS the sexy librarian. Always, always cast yourselves in the starring roles.

Following the librarian theme, one night ask her to wear her glasses to bed when you make love. Then, gradually get her to add a bit more – maybe putting her hair up as well, and adding pearls or a conservative outfit. If she agrees to dress up for you, surprise her with some sexy lingerie to wear underneath!

Eventually, you can work your way into a full-scale production!

The conversation you have about going that far, though, is an important one. Going whole-hog with role-playing takes some planning.

Assuming that she's been with you so far on this journey – and if you've taken your time, encouraged her and shown her an environment of trust and comfort, eventually she'll be right there with you – you can broach it as a wouldn't-it-be-cool-if type of thing.

Again, it should be fun and flirty – like I said before, playing dress-up is something that goes back to childhood, and there should be a child-like glee in getting everything ready. You can almost make it like you want to put on a play.

This is the time you bring up a safe word. Up until now, it's really only been the two of you, as yourselves, having sex while maybe talking dirty and dressing up. When you want to really assume these roles, there needs to be the ability to step out of character in a way that both of you understand.

Start off with something that takes a short amount of time, and then you can work up to lengthier play times.

By now, she might have a few role-playing ideas herself – so make sure to keep those lines of communication open, and see what she might have thought of all on her own!

Chapter 6: Porn: Watching It and Making Your Own

Talking about role play in terms of characters and scenes reminds me of another subject – recording your antics.

I'm sure this doesn't need to be said, but say it I will – DO NOT RECORD SEXUAL ACTS without explicit prior consent from your partner. Recording her having sex without her knowing is an enormous violation of the trust you've worked so hard to build.

- Don't think you can show it to her afterwards and she'll get turned on by it.

- Don't think you can hide it from her forever.

- And don't EVER think you can post it on the Internet or send it to even your closest friend.

If your fantasy is to see yourself having sex with her, then that's fine – but there is a way to go about doing this, and that is to include her every step of the way.

All women – even the most drop-dead beautiful women in the world – cringe when they see photos or videos of themselves. It's their first instinct, and it's a strong one. The same goes for anytime they're looking at themselves, even in a mirror – they are picking out their imperfections, and seeing where improvements can be made.

So, if you want to get your partner to the point where you're both watching her do the wild thing on camera, you've got to take it reeeeeeeally slowly.

Much of the same initial steps are similar to the exhibitionist fantasy we talked about a while back. You're going to want to get her comfortable with being seen, and being seen as beautiful in your eyes. This is really when you have to pull out all the stops in building up her confidence, ensuring that she trusts you, and making it about HER and you together.

Despite what you think, getting her to watch porn films with you is NOT the way to escalate this fetish. You're simply inviting her to compare herself to other women whose bodies she could never afford, nor afford to maintain. The focus, as always, has to be about how much SHE excites you.

If you've gotten her to talk about her own fantasies, make sure they happen. Reinforce how beautiful she is, how great it is that you two can be together in this free way, and how close you feel to her as you watch her let her inhibitions go.

Work up from darkness to candles to lights on. Slowly work in having sex in front of a mirror in the bedroom, in the bathroom mirror, or using nighttime interior windows. Make sure the light is always flattering to her, and remind

HOW TO GET HER TO...

her how beautiful she looks when she's having sex, how perfect her body is, how much you love seeing your bodies together.

This can and should be done with every possible bit of romance you can muster. Reinforce the connection you feel, witnessing the communion of your souls, her beauty.

Buy her gorgeous lingerie, and don't run and tear it off of her – ask if you can watch her in it for a while. Sexy pajamas and things she can wear around the house while not having sex will help her to feel beautiful. When purchasing lingerie, do everything in your power to make it COMFORTABLE as well as sexy. She's not going to get into it if she's tugging at seams and feeling like a tarted up whore.

Your next step is photographs. And this is where a serious conversation has to happen.

You MUST let her know EXACTLY what your intention is with the photographs. If you want to take them and have you look at them together afterwards as a one-time thing, let her know that – and delete the pictures together.

If you want to keep the pictures to view whenever you want, let her know every security measure you're taking – i.e., they will not be online, on a work computer, or anywhere where anyone other than you can get to them. Put them on a CD or DVD or data key, and have her keep it and get it from her when you want to look at them. Let her have final say in what pictures you can and can't keep.

Listen to her during this conversation, and make every effort to accommodate her requests.

This conversation, however, can also be a sexy one if done correctly. Viewing the pictures together can be an opportunity to lavish her with compliments. Let her know how hard it makes you to see her like that. If they are pictures of both of you, play up the romantic aspects of it.

Do not compare her to a porn star, super model or celebrity. This will make her compare herself to them, and she won't have the same reaction that you do. Just tell her she's beautiful, the most gorgeous creature that ever lived, you get the idea. Keep it about her.

Although unconventional, and it would require a tremendous amount of trust on her part, you could hire someone to take beautiful, artistic nude portraits of her or the two of you. I'm just throwing it out there. An excellent, trustworthy photographer with good post-production skills can do wonders for her ego and your fantasy.

Moving on to recording sex, this is where you can really make her a partner in your fantasy. You could do lots of tests for lighting and flattering poses, and then even edit the recording together and put music with it.

However, if at any time she balks, pull the plug – literally and figuratively – and drop the issue for a while. In the meantime, make sure there is lots of loving, romantic, media-free sex in the mix.

Watching Porn Together

Many guys who like mutual masturbation also enjoy watching porn with their wife or girlfriend. They can go hand in hand (yes, another pun)!

Simply put, porn freaks girls out.

- It makes them think of teenage boys' bedrooms, with stinky socks and old Farah Fawcett posters. And not in a good way.
- It makes them think of masturbating, which they might find gross.
- They find it degrading to women.
- They feel like you're comparing their bodies to porn stars' bodies.
- It makes them feel inadequate sexually.
- They get worried that the girls in the film were kidnapped and are doing this against their will or on drugs.
- They actually pay attention to, and thus find lacking, the plot, scenery, music, porn star noises and lighting.
- They are horrified by portrayals of sex they wouldn't do themselves – orgies, threesomes, lesbian sex, gang banging, fisting, etc.

The list goes on and on, but you get the basic idea – girls, as a rule, are not going to love it when you pop in a porn movie after dinner.

The best way to have her get over the stigma she attaches

to porn is to watch it for non-sexual entertainment purposes. Rent one as a joke – maybe while on vacation, on pay per view, if it's a rainy day. Make sure it's the lightest, worst produced porn you can find.

"Come on, it'll be hilarious! Grab some popcorn, we'll make fun of it like Mystery Science Theater." Crack jokes, laugh at the improbability of it all, get grossed out when she gets grossed out, just go with it. Try your best not to get turned on in any way.

Don't tell your buddies, and have it be like your fun little secret. Joke about it privately, maybe about how you consider yourselves film critics now, and you could have your own show reviewing porn for its artistic content.

Then, much later, maybe pick one up at the rental place – "Hey I saw this, I think this one might actually have a plot!" I'm not saying you should be renting one a week, but over time it can make her more comfortable to actually sit through a porn film with you.

Eventually, you'll want to watch one together that you find exciting -and let her know it, again in a light, joking way. "Wow, this one must be well made, because it's actually giving me a hard-on!" Don't try anything sexual, though.

Gradually you'll want to watch one that seriously turns you on, and talk during it – "This one is good." "This is seriously turning me on, what the hell?" "Um, I'm about to take you into the bedroom and ravish you, hope you don't mind!" Do just that, and you're letting her know that porn for you equals sex with her – remember, the focus should always come back to her.

Ask her what she does or doesn't like about the porn you've seen together, and listen to what she says, even if she's not talking about the sex parts – if she likes a certain plot, or a particular location, those can be important indicators that, although she's not saying it outright, she's enjoying the film.

Chapter 7: Going Beyond Missionary

Next, we're going to get into physical experimentation. This includes spanking, biting, anal play, use of sex toys and props, light bondage, and other naughty things that feature something being done to or with the body.

Mutual Masturbation

Girls have a very delicate relationship with masturbation, and one that will be completely foreign to you. There are very few girls who will admit to "rubbing one out" – and many have never even attempted it! I'll wait while that one sinks in.

Many guys like to see a girl touch herself, but girls will consider it too dirty, too embarrassing or just plain bad. But, there are some benefits – for one, there is no safer sex than masturbating. Second, it can give you a chance to learn what really turns her on. And finally, while it is a taboo, it's extremely harmless.

A touch of casual humor is the best way to get your gal to open up to the idea of masturbating in front of you, or mutual masturbating. Because it is usually such a private matter, and one that is extremely embarrassing for most women to even think about, let alone talk about or do, she needs to know that there is no shame in the touching game.

HOW TO GET HER TO...

The trick is to keep the language clean, at least at first. Is she taking forever in the bathroom? "Hey, are you touching yourself in there?" would be a light tease. If she's defensive, keep it light – "Hey, it's your loss if you're not! But if you are, hurry it up – we're going to be late!"

If she's looking like a hot mama one night, "Wow, you look great. How can you look that hot and not want to touch yourself? I sure would."

That kind of talk could lead to more "serious" discussions, in which it is best to feign absolute ignorance, if I may say so, in order to show her that you don't find anything wrong at all with masturbation. "Really? You don't masturbate? I thought everyone on earth masturbated. I don't know, it just seems like a perfectly normal thing for people to do."

If she gives you a line about girls in general not masturbating, don't buy it, but be easy – you don't want to get into a fight about it! "Aww, come on, that can't be true. Well, if it is true, that's a shame. Masturbating seems like a perfectly natural thing to do. I don't know why people are so embarrassed about it. I mean, I wouldn't walk into work and tell everyone, but between two people who are intimate, I don't see how it's any different than other things done in bed."

Mutual masturbation is also something that can be tried out during sex, if it is done gradually and always with romance and emotional connection as its focus.

When touching her body, slowly and gently take her hand in yours – almost like you want to hold her hand while you touch her. Follow along the contours of her body, the sides of her breasts, even her face. Don't go for vaginal touching until she is 100 percent comfortable with the kind of touching you're guiding her in now.

And again, focus on her, your connection, and her beauty. "Can you feel how soft your skin is?" "This is my favorite part of you." Get her involved in answering you.

If she starts with fake porn gasps, just plain old freezes up or pulls her hand away, back off and continue having sex. When you try again, make sure it's two or three times later, and start off very slowly.

Once she gets very, very used to both of you touching her, it might be a good time to play a game to have her touch herself without your guidance. I recommend the following, taking into account, obviously, that you've become enough advanced together as a couple in bed to try it. And, make it romantic as hell, not all about the sex.

Ask her to close her eyes, cover her eyes or wrap something VERY feminine – a scarf, or anything else of hers will do (I'll get into why a bit later when we cover light bondage). Then, take the condiment of your choice – chocolate sauce, whipped cream, honey (nothing too hot or too cold!) – and, with her eyes closed, ask her to touch the part of her body she wants you to put some of it (with the intent of you licking it off, naturally).

Then escalate the game by switching the rules – you can drip some onto her, and tell her she has to rub it in a bit before you'll lick it off. Be playful, and tell her she hasn't rubbed it in enough, or she missed some. You can see where that will lead, I hope.

The key is to always move slowly, make it romantic, and gradually escalate the touching until eventually, you're masturbating yourselves.

Love Bites

…But love shouldn't bleed! If you're wanting to bite your shy girl, or have her bite you, it should always be light and playful. There are several elements of biting that can freak out a less experimental girl:

- You might leave a mark on her that someone will see.
- It reminds her of hickeys, and high school, yuck.
- Ouch! You're hurting her.
- She might be afraid of hurting you or doing it "wrong."
- It can be seen as an aggressive act.
- It can be seen as just plain weird.

The beginning stages of biting should be done during non-sexual times, and in a very playful way. "You look so yummy, I just want to eat you up!" And nuzzle her shoulder.

Have her feed you, and keep her fingers in your mouth, sucking on them and then lightly biting them.

Very light, playful wrestling or horsing around can include a little nip or two.

While making out, slightly bite her lip, her ear. Stay away from the neck, she'll scream about hickeys. The neck is only ok if you quickly run down from her ear to her collarbone, in a kind of funny "nom nom nom" way, never using teeth.

While in bed, kiss her all over until she gets very used it and/or turned on by it. Then, in each place you choose, kiss, kiss longer, and then nip lightly. Move right onto the next place – you don't want her to think you're going to dig in.

Once she is comfortable with that, you can move onto more intimate parts to bite lightly – ass cheeks, inner thighs, breasts. Be VERY careful around her nipples – while some girls like a bit of tweaking or biting, some have extremely sensitive nipples and even a light suck might make her yelp in pain.

Finally, once she's on board, you can gradually increase the strength of the bites to your pleasure. Don't break any skin, and if she protests, softly say sorry, kiss the spot you hurt, and move on.

If you want her to bite you, game time in nice. Do a tit-for-tat touching and kissing game, with you kissing her on a spot, and she kissing you on the same spot on your body with the same "force." Gradually work up to biting, and encourage her to bite harder if you want – just make sure you never do it more than she wants to her body!

HOW TO GET HER TO...

Spanking (And Doin' It Doggy-Style)

Like biting, spanking can be seen as an aggressive act, so it should start off light and playful. A smack on the ass while you're in the kitchen making dinner together can start things off right.

But, unlike biting, there really is no way to ease into spanking – you either are spanking, or you're not. So, unlike almost all the other advice in this book, I'm going to go ahead and say that spanking just needs to be tried.

Your best time is, of course, while having sex doggy-style. If even this is a little too forward-thinking for your ladylove, then it is something you can work up to gradually – but it means that spanking is way, way off in the future.

Giving her a sexy full back massage is the best way to get her facing the right way, especially if you're super-romantic about it. Let it be all about her pleasure, keeping the focus on her and her body.

Fingering her while she's in a massage position, after working your way up her legs, should be incredibly erotic for her at this point. Especially if you've already given her orgasms using your hands, she will be into it. And, being into it, her natural physical instinct will be to arch her back so that area is more open for you to explore.

You really want to get her going while she's in this position, and almost close to orgasm. While continuing to play with her with one hand, slide your other hand under

GOING BEYOND MISSIONARY

her pelvic/belly area and guide her up to the doggy position.

This is when you're going to enter her from behind – and when it is absolutely crucial that you keep at least one hand in physical contact with her. It's important because the number one thing that women don't like about this position is the possibility of your going in the wrong hole – which is a whole other area we'll talk about in a bit – and if they can't see what's going on back there, and they're with their ass in the air and don't feel your immediate presence, they're going to get nervous and think you don't know which hole to put it in, either. Game over!

It's best if you use the hand you're fingering her with to simultaneously guide yourself into her – then she will know you're doing it right.

Start off slowly, rhythmically, and follow her movements. Work your way up to orgasm – hey, for her as well! In this position, you can always reach around for a bit of clitoral stimulation. If you as a couple are not familiar with this position, it's important to let her take the lead in moving the two of you around.

If your penis comes out, again guide it back in using your hand, and start slowly again. It might suck for both of you, but you don't want to be slamming away and have it go in the wrong hole. And trust me – neither does she.

If you're into watching your penis thrust in and out of her, kneel fully up, hold both her hips steady and do it slowly, for the same reason as above. As you speed up toward orgasm, keep it close to her, with your pelvis up against her body as much as possible. Near-orgasm wrong-hole mistakes are the most common.

Once you're comfortable as a couple doing it doggy-style, you can start off with caressing, then rubbing her ass while in that position. Do that a couple of times until she gets used to your touch on her ass.

When you first attempt spanking, do it LIGHTLY and JUST ONCE.

Next time, you can do it a couple of times, but still lightly.

Ease back into just rubbing her ass during doggy-style sex.

It's best to wait until she is in the full swing of a doggy-style session until you crack one on her ass. Again, JUST ONCE. She might cry out, and it might sound like she liked it – but you probably caught her mid-gasp, and trust me, there will be a bit of a surprise OUCH in that yelp as well.

The next few times you have sex doggy-style, spank her again, just once.

Work up to full spanking slowly, one smack at a time. If she protests, STOP and say you're sorry, but her ass is just so hot you couldn't help yourself. Then back off the spanking and work your way back up.

Anal!

You thought Sex And The City was never good for anything except her escalating wardrobe bills – but as it turns out, you might have Carrie and friends to thank for women being a lot more open to anal sex than ever before.

Pun intended, of course.

Anal sex has always been the ultimate taboo, or at best, part of a backwards mentality among some cultures that think anal sex is the way to get some good loving while saving your "real virginity" until marriage.

I'm not going to get into that whole discussion, you can thank your lucky stars, or else we'll be here until the end of time. But, there has been a stigma attached to what is considered the ultimate slutty act that even SATC hasn't been able to overcome entirely.

But, it's not just the slut factor. To put it bluntly, it's about the poop.

Overall, girls are about 4,000 percent more meticulous about hygiene and cleanliness than guys. There are girls who have never farted – in private, let alone in front of anyone – and there are girls who have never looked in the bowl after taking a dump.

Girls think butts are dirty, period. And there is no amount of logic that is going to make them see otherwise. So if you want your ladylove to welcome you through the back door, it's going to take you some time.

HOW TO GET HER TO...

There are some non-negotiable rules about anal:

1. Use lubrication, and by that, I mean go into a store and buy real lube. Not spit, not olive oil, not massage oil. LUBE.

2. Never go ass-to-mouth. No blowjobs after anal sex, no kissing after rimming, no eating her out after rimming her.

3. Never go ass-to-vagina. Once you're in, you're in to win.

Some world-class listening is needed on your part in order to have anything to do with her ass. If she feels bloated, if she's complaining about constipation, if she complains about anything remotely related to food consumption or digestion, it's off. Also, never try it after she's eaten, for your own sake.

Like doggy-style above, my advice might sound strange at first – but frankly, there really is no fun, creative, delicate or otherwise romantic way to tell her you want to have anal sex with her. It's going to take a lot of slow, gradual escalation to get to the point where she feels comfortable with it.

The first few times you've both assumed the position, bring her to orgasm by fingering her, or do it doggy style. She needs to understand you know your way around that area. Doggy-style needs to become a regular, almost "boring" part of your bedroom repertoire. Keep the focus on her, and let her know that you think you love how she moves under you in that position.

Any action near the anus should first be done with your fingers. You can start the same way as doggy-style, with long, romantic massages. However, it's best if maybe you take a steamy shower together, so she knows she's as clean as she's going to get once you start playing back there. She doesn't need to know why you want to shower with her; she'll figure it out soon enough.

Start by caressing lightly – like, butterfly-kisses-lightly – her ass cheeks and the crack of her ass. Keep moving back to fingering her vaginal area.

Over the next couple of sessions, whether during sex or in a massage situation, massage her ass using a bit more pressure, pushing with your palm a bit along her ass crack. While fingering her, move further and further back toward her anus, but don't enter.

Then, work up to fingering the outside of her anus, massaging it straight-fingered, with no hint of penetration. Pay attention to her reaction. While I'm generally not a fan of continuing after she protests, unless she really freaks out, calm her down while continuing to massage the anus area without penetration. She's worried you're going to pop it in there, so let her get used to you NOT doing that.

When it comes time to penetrating her anus with your finger – and that's singular, that's ONE finger – there are a few things to remember:

HOW TO GET HER TO...

1. Make sure she is physically relaxed and in a comfortable position before you try it.

2. Lubricate your forefinger and middle finger with her vaginal juices, or have some lube nearby. You don't want to be going in there dry.

3. Make sure your nails are clipped short and smooth, with no hangnails or jagged edges.

4. You can't go back to fingering her vaginal area, so make sure she's either already had an orgasm or that you're willing to completely switch up your sexual position if she freaks out. Note, switching positions does NOT mean reverting to doggy-style – best is straight missionary sex. She won't be into doggy-style because she's going to think you're going to try anal with your penis, which one hopes is substantially larger than the finger you just used.

5. If she does freak out, there should be lots of soothing talk and cuddling involved. You've just penetrated a brand new area of her body, and she didn't like it – give her a comfort zone.

Your fore or middle finger works best, as you can massage her ass cheeks a bit while you're going in. You want to develop a rhythm she can rely on, and do it for a while without going back to her vaginal area so she gets used to the idea of your finger being where it is. Gradually increase the pressure of your finger a bit at a time, and when it comes time to enter her with your finger, slow the rhythm down a bit but keep it consistent.

You want to enter her as slowly, lovingly and gently as you would with your penis into her vagina during a magically romantic session of making passionate, soul-searing love. Seriously.

Keep a slow, consistent rhythm going, but don't start going in and out with your finger – keep it where it is, and use the ebbing motion to simply pulse your finger, and the flowing motion to incrementally move it further into her anus by MILLIMETERS. Really, really slowly. Achingly slowly.

If she does freak out, don't snap your finger out of her anus. Keep your voice soft, say, "OK, honey," place your other hand gently on the small of her back, and ease your finger out slowly. Do NOT get out of bed to clean your hand; have a washcloth or wipe ready, but do not leave her there after you've just penetrated her ass. Kiss her, hold her, and be very gentle and loving with her; if she indicates she'd still like to have sex, make it vanilla.

Once finger penetration is a comfortable addition to sex, your only immediate goal is to work your one finger further inside. Way down the line is two fingers. You don't want to do more than that.

Entering with two fingers should be done at the same time. Don't get one in there and then try to squeeze the other one in – you run the risk of tearing her sensitive skin.

HOW TO GET HER TO...

To get her used to the idea of your penis being a part of the action, as she gets more comfortable with your fingers all the way inside her, you want to make sure the hand inside her is facing palm up, so that if you bent your hand you'd be cupping her ass. While keeping an ever-steady rhythm, and with your hand cupping her ass, move your body lengthwise alongside hers, with yourself partly on top of her, and using your rhythmic movements, get both of your bodies into the rhythm of lovemaking.

Keep it slow!

Do this several times until this, too becomes a normal feature of sex for the two of you. Always follow up this move with romantic, gentle vaginal sex as vanilla as you can take it. Lots of kissing, cuddling, soft words.

When it's penis time, you'll want to do a little finger play at first, and get her comfortable. By this time, you should have already entered lube into the sexual routine of this position, perhaps even using it for doggy-style sex, so she is used to the pause while you put it on and the sensation of it against her skin. (Please, on behalf of women everywhere and also your penis, make sure the lube isn't super cold.)

While you're doing the kind of fingering/cupping/humping thing, tell her want to "be inside" her "like this." If she says no, say O.K. and drop it.

One day, she's going to let you do it. Like I've said much earlier in this book, don't act like she just gave you a puppy. Use all your restraint and keep your movements calm and gentle. Remember to take your fingers out of her SLOWLY, don't snap them out.

Like you've been doing doggy-style, ease her body into position and use your finger to massage the anus, gradually and slowly replacing it with your penis. Keep your rhythmic movements consistent, because she's freaking out and tensing up right now – and you really, really need her as relaxed as possible.

Let the tip of your penis push against her anus for several rounds of rhythmic movements, and ssslllooowwwlllyyy ease it in. Slow rhythm, slow penetration, slow, slow, slow. Rub her back, massage her hips, everything slow and romantic so she stays relaxed.

Sometimes, a girl's anus can make a farting noise when your penis or even your fingers are inside her. No giggling, no jokes, no talking about it afterwards.

From now until you achieve orgasm, you have to keep it slow. It will take you a while to get fully inside her, and let yourself just kind of be in there a while before you start going for the gold. And don't forget, no matter how flaccid you become after orgasm, you've gotta come out just as slowly as you went in.

Don't forget to check and make sure the condom came out with you.

Have a washcloth or small hand towel nearby to give a quick wipe, and then cuddle the shit out of her. Lay there for as long as she wants. Only when she's either asleep or has gotten up out of bed do you do so as well.

Do not react to any traces of feces anywhere until you are alone in the bathroom. Get washed up really, really, really well, because she's going to freak out and never let you do it again if she smells even a scintilla of poop anywhere near you or the bed. Even if you want to shower with her after, clean yourself up first in private.

Either flush the condom or wrap it in lots of toilet paper before chucking it in the trash. And, you're in charge of cleanup – wash the outside of the lube bottle and put it away, and either hand wash and dry before putting in the laundry, or offer to wash an entire load yourself along with whatever hand towel or wash cloth you used while having anal sex. Check that there are no poop drips or stains wherever you had sex.

And that's how to get your wife or girlfriend to have anal sex!

Your Butt
First off, let me say that there is absolutely NOTHING weird, gay, bad, wrong or abnormal in men wanting to have their ass played with during sex. And do you know why? Because that is where the prostate lives – and the prostate is a one-way ticket to Orgasm City.

And if your partner understands this, it becomes a much less taboo thing to do. The same basic gross-out factor applies for women, so anytime you want to try this you'll have to make sure she knows that you've just taken a shower and scrubbed up good!

There's really no gradual way for her to get into the idea unless you first tell her what it is you want her to do. After that's been made clear, then you can suggest starting with a massage, and make appreciative sounds the closer she gets to the prize.

If your girl is heavy into long manicured talons, you're going to need to warn her to be extra careful – or, have her wear a condom over her finger while she's back there.

You also might want to go for a bit of manscaping if you're a hairy bear back there – it might go a long way in her agreeing to go along with you on this. At the very least, she'll know you're serious about it!

Unlike anal penetration on her, when it's done on you you're going to want to take care of the cleanup as soon as humanly possible. Have wipes or a trip to the bathroom ready to administer to whatever parts touched your anus. Don't give her time to examine her fingers. Then, big hugs and kisses and cuddling afterward – she's not used to penetrating a man in any way, and it might be an uncomfortable feeling for her emotionally.

Rimming

The same basic rules apply for rimming as for all other anal play, and should not be attempted with a sexually inexperienced girl until she's well familiar with you being in her ass area, or vice-versa.

You want to work up from massaging and penetrating the area with your fingers or penis, to working kissing her ass cheeks into your routine. Get closer and closer to the anus, and if she tenses, back off and kiss her in other places on her body that she loves.

Remember, once you succeed in rimming her, you're going to need to thoroughly wash out your mouth before kissing her or her other pretty parts.

Props and Sex Toys: Part I

A woman who owns sex toys is a woman who is serious about her sexual pleasure. If you were dating this kind of woman, you probably wouldn't need this book. So, let's see if we can convince your own woman to be a babe in Toyland!

Again, you owe a debt of gratitude to Sex and the City for even being able to broach this subject with your ladylove. And, thanks to the Internet, you now can browse and purchase even the most naughty toys and props from the privacy of your own home – and keep your accountant or nosy doorman out of your bedroom proclivities as well, with boring-sounding company names on your statements and excellent, discreet packaging.

Toys of any kind are all about playing, which is the foremost thing to keep in mind whenever you're dealing with sex toys.

As always, you want to start off slow here – but there are a couple of things you can do sooner rather than later to introduce the idea of props and sex toys into your bedroom activities. Let's discuss some of them now!

Did you know your home is already full of sex toys? It's true! If you're able to be spontaneous enough, you can get her used to many different types of stimulation from things other than you and your body. The key is to be safe – nothing that can get lodged up there, nothing that can be broken easily, nothing sharp, and nothing too long.

Have sex on the washing machine during the spin cycle, or on the kitchen counter while the dishwasher is running. She should be sitting up, and you should be standing.

For other locations and with the introduction of household objects, the focus should be on pleasuring her – lots of oral sex, massages, fingering should be a part of this. Don't be pounding away at her and then switch it up with an object – it will seem aggressive and invasive to her.

The kitchen has plenty more to offer as well – wine bottles, ice cubes, chocolate syrup, whipped cream, and even vegetables can be used in the heat of passion. Sounds strange, I know – but it can be done in a way that can be fun and titillating for her.

Start off with condiments in the bedroom, licking them off her body. Whipped cream is best for this, and you can spray it right into her vagina – not too far, though – and then lick it out.

To get a bit more adventurous, get her up on the kitchen

counter and start pleasing her with your hands or your mouth. Then, reach over and gently start pleasuring her with whatever object is handy (keep it safe, please!).

A sensuous bath or shower might do the trick as well – bottles of hair conditioner, the handle of a back scrubber, or even a small bar of soap can be played with near and in her vagina.

The living room can yield candles, remotes or decorative objects. Have fun, be inventive – just keep it slow, passionate and about her pleasure. And be safe!

Back in the bedroom, blindfolding or extremely light bondage can be introduced with scarves and other accessories of hers. If your girl is especially shy about this, take care to use her things – I wouldn't even use a necktie of yours until she's comfortable with using her own stuff.

You can even buy "funny" things for this, without them being considered sex toys – a feather boa, say, or cutesy ribbons are good, playful examples. I'll say again, Halloween or theme parties are a great excuse to buy some of these props, and then have them become a normal part of the house and therefore less threatening or taboo.

"Gag" gifts can be a harmless way to get the idea of toys and fun into the discussion, too. Edible underwear, flavored condoms, pubic hair dye and other things can help establish an element of play that makes the addition of toys seem like a logical progression. I'd hold off on fake handcuffs – even the kind that have pink fur on them – until you've established a routine of trust and comfort with any kind of restraint play.

In terms of "real" sex toys – vibrators, cock rings, dildos, anal beads, butt plugs, etc. – recommend a party line of "well, we've got one now, let's try it and see what it does!" It's almost like watching porn together in that the whole time, you're mindful of the fact that other people get off on it, and you're curious to find out why.

A bachelor party can be a good excuse to bring home a sex toy – you can say they were given out as party favors, perhaps. On the other end of the spectrum, Valentine's Day gifts can include a sex toy for her or both of you, as a kind of gag gift that you just happened to see as you were out shopping for her, or that you had read about in all the press leading up to the holiday.

It's worth saying again that fun, curiosity and light playing can make the introduction of sex toys and props into your sex life something that becomes a sharing time, as opposed to, "I want to do this thing, and I'm convincing you to do it too."

Sex toy usage, and the types of sex toys themselves, can gradually escalate to strap-on dildos, customized dildos, sex swings, whips, full bondage gear, and a whole galaxy of other items. The key, as always, is to be safe, have a safe word, take it slowly and keep the focus on sharing these experiences from a mutual basis of curiosity and fun.

Props and Sex Toys: Part II

There are some kinds of sexual experimentation that, while including props and sex toys, are on a little bit of a more serious level than what we've just discussed. You want to establish a long, healthy, safe, loving and trustful sexual relationship, with lots of different kinds of experimentation, before moving onto this level – and even then, it's important to move at a very slow pace and be receptive to her reactions, comments or complaints.

This is also a good time to go back to talking. And talking. And talking. You want to be as open as possible with each other, and not shy away from having frank discussions about sex, sex roles, and experimentation. And, you're going to want to give as good as you get – try the things she wants to do, and keep the discussion going.

Chapter 8: Taking It Up a Notch

Right now we're going to get into more involved sexual experimentations, and how to ease your partner into finding enjoyment in sharing them with you.

Gender Play

Gender play is just what it sounds like – where one or both partners assume the character or identity of the opposite gender during sex. This can be achieved through verbal means or, depending on the combination, with the help of clothing, props and/or sex toys.

For instance, a man could perhaps shave his body hair, wear women's lingerie or don a wig and makeup. A woman could dress like a man, and/or wear a strap-on dildo. Or, one or the other of you could simply adjust your voice and engage in dirty talk.

This doesn't necessarily mean that both genders must reverse, either. You can engage in homosexual experimentation through gender play, too.

While the role-playing we have gone over in this book so far is considered more of a playful bedroom pastime, gender play reaches a bit deeper into the psyche and literally turns the relationship upside down. In fact, many couples' counselors suggest gender play in the bedroom as one method in getting partners to understand the feelings of each other.

However, role-playing is a logical foundation for gender play, and should definitely be used in the progression into gender play. Again, Halloween and theme parties can come in handy for this, to keep it fun and non-sexual at first.

Gender play, especially for those who are not particularly experimental, or have only recently started experimenting with sex, can be a significant experience. No matter how equal and trusting your relationship is, assuming a role that is fundamentally different than one you've been used to for your entire life can awaken a whole host of confusing thoughts and feelings, and can break open many of the assumptions and prejudices you might not have even known you held.

But all of the seriousness aside, gender play may be something that can bring your relationship to a whole new level, both in and out of the bedroom. And, for many who enjoy it, it can also be wildly erotic.

Some important things to keep in mind for gender play:

Unless the agreed-upon parameters of your play involve spending non-sexual time as the opposite gender, it can be best, especially at first, to keep it confined to the bedroom.

In any case, make sure you mark the specific beginning and end of your gender playtime.

Be mindful of the psychological ramifications of a man being penetrated by a woman, for both of you. This is done through the use of a strap-on dildo. The same basic rules apply for "pegging," as it is called, as for anal sex in the reverse.

However, you might feel like having "traditional" sex before or afterward, and that is fine. However, if this has not been worked out beforehand, I advise you to not be aggressive with your girl when getting back to penetrating her – it can lead to a type of ugly "tit for tat" that can erode a relationship.

The parameters set by the two of you for gender play should be clear not only for when it starts and ends, but how far to take your roles. Above, I recommended keeping it confined to the bedroom, because there are two facets to gender play – the sexual component, and the relationship component. You want to make sure that you're not using gender play as a way to be passive-aggressive in working out whatever relationship problems you have, unless you're under the supervision of a counselor or psychiatric advisor.

The parameters are also important for going too far sexually, and like with other things we've talked about, a safe word is absolutely mandatory for gender play. If the safe word is used by either of you, it's important to leave the bedroom, change back into your normal clothes, and let some time pass before perhaps discussing what element was uncomfortable for either of you.

Just remember – gender play and other role reversals are used by loving, heterosexual couples every day. In no way does wanting to experiment with gender roles signify that you are homosexual. Both you and your partner need to truly grasp this fact in order for there to be uninhibited play.

Sissification

Gender play can be taken to an even more intense level with sissification – which is when your woman treats you like a lesbian lover. Sissification is a form of female domination, in as far as the biological woman takes the lead in the scenario by teaching the man how to look, act, and sexually treat her more like a woman would.

Again, parameters must be agreed to before embarking on sissification. You need to decide whether it's just bedroom play, or if it will extend to, say, wearing panties every day, answering to a female name and restricting the amount of penetrative sex you have.

It's not for sissies, no pun intended. This pushes the envelope on gender play.

You'll want to start out with a lot of naughty talk for this one, and you're going to want to avoid penetrative sex during it, which obviously misses the point. A good topic is her own body – "Your body is so beautiful, your breasts are so beautiful, what does it feel like to have breasts? I'd love to have a vagina for a day, just to feel what it's like," etc.

Sissification can also be a broachable subject if your partner has talked about wanting to experiment with other women, or has wondered about what it is like to be a lesbian, sexually speaking. By you assuming the role of a female, you can encourage her to live out this fantasy without having to go outside the relationship.

Female Domination

While each person stays in their biological roles, female domination takes gender roles to an extreme reversal. Like sissification, female domination can become a lifestyle, in which her domination over you affects every part of your life, or it can be reserved simply for bedroom activities.

So, you know the drill: Talking, parameters, safe word, slow escalation, and more talking. And, again, there is absolutely nothing wrong with you or your sexuality for wanting to explore this part of your relationship.

It is important for you to know how far you want to take it, so that you can lead her to that point. If you want her to direct all sex play, it requires a different road than, say, if you want to lick her shoes clean and eat out of a dog bowl.

Despite this being an advanced form of sexual experimentation, it can be easier to get your partner involved by dint of the fact that it involves her being in a dominant role. You might want to start out with a type of "Queen for a Day" scenario, in which you tell her that you will do anything she says for a day, a weekend, and even building up to a week.

You can make it just for the bedroom, or extend it to household chores, massages on demand, how, where and what you eat, and other ideas. Again, it all depends on what kind and what level of female domination you're looking to achieve.

This might be a good type of fetish to research together. There is plenty of information available, from books to guides to documentaries, and professional dominatrices in your area can teach your partner how to do it right.

A popular activity for female domination is the creampie – where the man eats out his own semen after having ejaculated inside of his partner. This probably doesn't need a lot of prior discussion, but if she gets grossed out by your doing it, you can simply explain that it excites you.

Another one is a leash fetish (also known as a collar and lead in British English). This is where the man is led around by the woman on a leash, either walking or on all fours. This is also connected to being the "pet," in which the man eats out of a feeding bowl and is forced to perform his bodily functions as a pet would.

Teasing and Denial

A popular form of female domination is to deny the man orgasms. While it might seem nearly impossible to be able to talk about this with your partner – "O.K., now tease me until I can't take it anymore, and then tell me not to come" – it can be achieved through, again, a slow escalation.

Gradually prolonged foreplay is the best starting point to this type of experimentation, and will introduce the "tease" element into the scenario. This might be seen less a fetish and more like a rollicking good time to her, since most women complain about their men not giving enough foreplay!

If you're into teasing and denying orgasms for both of you, this can be achieved by not only prolonging the foreplay, but also by stopping at a certain point with a (followed-through) promise of completion at a later point. Emphasize how good it will feel the longer you wait – but it's crucial you do earn her trust by coming through with the goods.

If it is you who wants to be denied orgasm, again, it's usually perfectly O.K. with the ladies! You'll want to make sure to pleasure her, though, and to guide her through what it is you want to achieve with denial games. For example, let her give you a blowjob – and then right before you come, pull her up to you for some kissing, so you're denying it yourself. Eventually, you can ask her to "not let you" come by stopping on her own when she feels you are ready to explode.

If you're into denying her orgasms, well, I don't recommend trying this one AT ALL until you've made clear to her what it is you want from her, or else you're going to have one seriously pissed off lady on your hands. It's more important for this than any other denial scenario that you let her know when she will be having an orgasm, so she doesn't turn to auto-stimulation – or a lover.

Chastity Belt

Your final goal in wanting to be sissified, dominated or denied sexual pleasure is the chastity belt. Chastity belt "training," as it tends to be called, is a long-term scenario in which your partner literally locks up your penis and "releases" you only when she deems fit.

Don't worry – it's completely safe, sanitary and they even make plastic versions so you won't get called out in the airport security line! And there is a ton of information available on prostate milking, penis cleaning and other health issues, so you won't be completely neglected.

Chastity belts give her full dominance over your sexual nature, and really should not be a part of your dominance fetish until your partner is 400 percent comfortable in her role. And, as with female domination, a bit of research done together can help you set parameters and understand the "game" better, so there is a mutual feeling of satisfaction in the changes you're making to your relationship.

Chastity belt training requires a tremendous amount of trust and a long-term commitment to the process, so it isn't to be undertaken lightly. However, there is a silver lining in all of this – if you are successful in getting your woman to harness you into a chastity belt, I think we can safely assume that she's no longer shy about sexual experimentation!

Bondage and Discipline

Chips, dip, chains, whips – no doubt you've seen a million different portrayals on TV and in the movies of BD, as it's called in the fetish community; but like some of the other extreme domination scenarios we've been discussing, it requires a serious commitment and a hell of a lot of trust, as well as a healthy dose of sexual experimentation experience and a strong commitment to safety.

One other important component of bondage and discipline is the research and the preparation. Therefore, for the purposes of this book I'm not going to get into all the possible activities that come under the BD category; we're going to talk more about expressing these desires to your mate, getting her on board and what you can do to start experimenting.

There are a ton of books, guides, and communities online and off that can walk you through the particulars of BD, and can take a lot of the stigma and/or mystery out of it.

In addition to reading-style research, I highly recommend looking into consulting a professional dominatrix who can show you the ropes (there I go again with my puns!). There is a particular mindset and a specific set of guidelines that go in to the proper execution of a bondage and discipline scenario. And, putting a face to the fetish in many cases can put your lady at ease, believe it or not.

When talking it over with your mate, you want to emphasize a few things:

- Research and explain the connection between pleasure and pain. She's not going to want to hurt you if she doesn't understand why you want her to.

- We talked about light bondage in the Sex Toys section, but BD brings out the serious ties that bind. You'll want to do a lot of playful scarf/necktie/flirty materials tying up before you bust open the rope.

- In terms of restricting movements, whether with ropes, chains, handcuffs or wearable items, this again will need a lot of explanation in a school-lecture fashion. There are many reasons behind wanting to be restricted, and it's important that she's aware of them so she doesn't think you're just plain off your rocker – or that you're not interested in returning the favor.

- However, if you are wanting to perform BD on your partner, this too will need explaining. You want to emphasize the erotic aspects of it, and that it is not in any way, shape or form connected to how you feel about her in the context of your relationship.

- If you do succeed in doing this, as usual reinforce your tender side, and let her know how much it means to you, too. Not every girl in the world would do this for her guy, even after he employs my techniques!

Male Force and Domination

We've been talking a lot about female domination, but both women and men have male domination fantasies that can be realized as well. However, due to the fact that the overwhelming majority of sex-related crime in the world is committed by men, it's a subject that must be treated with the utmost discretion, trust, care and understanding.

Male domination is an especially sensitive subject if you're trying to get your partner to play along. You've really got to take it easy with this one. And you thought safe words were important for the other things we've talked about? Well, get ready – they are never more important than in male domination scenarios. Sorry, guys, but that's just the way of the world.

If your partner has been raped, assaulted or sexually abused in the past, this game is off the table. Don't even think about bringing it up.

If you have any faithful pets that are avid protectors of their masters, you'll want to make sure they are nowhere near the area you'll be playing in.

Any male domination experimentation MUST be done with the FULL CONSENT of your wife or girlfriend BEFORE you lay a finger on her. There is no negotiation on this point – no matter how much of a trusting relationship you have, no matter how much of a milquetoast you are in real life, even if she would swear on a stack of Bibles that she is 100 percent sure you would never hurt her in any way, there is no busting this kind of move without her agreeing to it beforehand.

This kind of sexual game cannot, under any circumstances, be done spontaneously or incorporated on the fly during another sex game. Even if you have successful male domination experiences under your belts, it is imperative that you separate those times from your normal lovemaking or other kinds of experimentation (although male domination can be incorporated into role-playing scenarios, which we'll discuss in a moment).

I'm going to start at the end on this one: After you've finished any sex involving male domination or force play, make sure there is ample time to spend being very gentle, loving and tender toward your partner. It reinforces the fantasy element of what you've just done as well as the trust factor in your sexual relationship. It will also help you come out of what can be a very explosive and potentially addictive role for you.

If this is a fantasy she'd like to see carried out, it's important to encourage her to talk about it; to stress that it is perfectly normal for women to have home-invasion, rape or other kinds of male force sexual fantasies; and to express to her your understanding that this does NOT mean she wants to be sexually assaulted in real life, by you or anyone else.

When watching news stories about assault, portrayals in film of sex crimes, or even if a hot handyman comes over to fix the bathroom pipes, don't be a dick and make a joke referring to her fantasy. I'm sure you wouldn't dream of it, but I had to put it out there. It's very important that her fantasy stays in the comfort zone of your trusting, loving relationship and not connected to any real-life, dangerous scenarios.

Once more about the safe word – male domination or force play involves your partner saying no, fighting you off or even trying to escape from your grasp. It's part of the excitement, because these games start with her begging you to stop, and then begging you NOT to stop as she becomes aroused by being penetrated against her will.

So, understandably, you're not going to actually stop when she says, "Stop" or "No" or even "Ouch, quit it!" That's why a safe word that has nothing to do with your scenario needs to be agreed upon – as is the fact that you're to stop immediately and hold her gently, with no judgments.

What you DO want to do is elicit from her exactly what her fantasy entails beforehand, so that you can work together in building up to making it happen. Because force fantasies are pretty on the edge, you'll want to be experienced in a lot of non-forceful role playing, depending on what she has in mind.

Let's say she wants you to be a high-school athlete who takes her, the mousy schoolgirl, behind the stadium for a quickie. You could start by wearing a team jersey, and give her some books to hold or maybe a plaid skirt to wear, and act out some short improvisational scenes that don't involve sex in any way.

Or, say she has a fantasy about being ravished by a delivery guy or a handyman who comes to the house. Wear a shirt and pants of the same color and get a clipboard, or carry your toolbox or a pizza box. You can change your voice or your accent, to make yourself seem different and to make it as real as possible within her comfort zone.

To reinforce the fantasy aspect, maybe have her wear an apron or something she normally doesn't wear around the house – or even just a towel, like she was fresh from a shower! Think of ways to make it more sexy, and less assault-y.

HOW TO GET HER TO...

You want to collaborate on the scenarios, and establish the characters as routine in your own way. Then, you can escalate to the point where you're engaging in forced-sex game playing.

Again, depending on your woman and her fantasy, this can be quick or slow. Is it being forced to have sex for the first time by a high school love, or is it someone who barges into the house and throws her on the bed? After it's over and you've been tender with her – or whenever the time seems right – ask her what she liked and didn't like, and how you can improve on it. This will go a long way in reinforcing to her that you understand it was, in fact, just a game.

Now, if it is you who wants this scenario, it's a whole other ball of wax.

Your best bet is to start out with hot, steamy, quickie sex that can be a bit rough and that comes after a very playful, romantic, flirty evening. Play it up on the way home, so she knows what's coming – with dirty whispers, ear nibbling, a discreet make-out session. Then, as soon as you get in the door, grab her and go at it – be ravenous, and very much into pleasing her. If she balks – "Stop, I have to pee, let me go to the bathroom first!" – be nice about it, stop, and gauge her mood when she returns before starting up again.

And don't ruin or tear her clothing. She'll be pissed off at you.

You want the idea of consensual force to become a passionate, romantic, routine part of your sexual repertoire as a couple. This will get her used to the idea of you "taking her" in the heat of the moment, and of your physical strength – without the fear factor.

You can broach the subject of force play by referring to these times, and saying that you wish you could be a delivery man or handyman who would just barge in and ravish her. Again, pay close attention to her reactions – they will tell you a lot. A great deal of objective talking should be done before bringing up your fantasy.

As for actually trying it out after she's willing to do it, the same rules apply as above.

Seriously, though, just be careful – this can really mess with a girl's mind if not executed properly, and could damage your relationship.

Chapter 9: Exploring the Fringe of All Things Kinky

We've covered all the major, "common" kinks and fetishes that might interest you and your ladylove and how you might go about sharing them and making them a part of your sexual repertoire. I really hope that I've given you some insight into the literally exciting world of sexual experimentation!

As you explore this new world, particularly while doing additional research – which I sincerely hope you do, because we've only scratched the surface here – you might come across some of the thousands of lesser-known kinks and fetishes, some of which are very unusual indeed.

Some of them might titillate you. Most of them will probably confuse you. Many of them you'll find on the Internet, which is exactly where they should stay. And, there are a few that simply make you wonder how they came to be, and where fans of them managed to find each other.

I was once at a gathering with fellow sexperts (nothing kinky, calm down) and we tried to think of something for which there could not possibly be a fetish. After much conversation (and laughter), we came up with one: knitting. We couldn't believe there could possibly be anyone who fetishized knitting.

Well, lo and behold, not only is there a knitting fetish – there are two subgroups! One fetishizes women in the act of knitting, and the other is more into women wearing knitted clothing. Go figure.

While fetishes are erotic or sexual in nature, not a few of them do not involve any sex at all; others involve simply masturbating; and still others require lots of play culminating in some kind of sexual act.

Just for the fun of it, let's take a look at some of them, shall we?

Remember – DON'T JUDGE.

Water Sports and Scat Play

These terms do not imply yachting or jazz singing. They are, respectively, a woman urinating or defecating on or near her partner. This kink is overwhelmingly performed by the female for the male, although some rare exceptions do apply; but these two kinks are pretty much reserved for female domination and worship.

I'm not going to lie to you; this is a pretty extreme fetish for someone whose partner is not particularly experimental. You're going to have to get her into a routine of kinky sex before even broaching this subject in any way.

Your best backup for this one are the facts. Urine is sterile, so it's not going to harm you (unless she has eaten or drunk something you're allergic to). And, you'll gain a ton of points by thinking ahead for clean up – the best place to first try this out is the shower, by far. Some couples that are really into it will lay down plastic or purchase rubber sheets for their adventures.

If even a willing partner is willing to give it a shot, but has trouble performing bathroom functions in front of anyone, the key is LOTS of water (not other kinds of beverages, as it tends to give an odor to the urine). She'll be practically begging to pee.

Any kind of sexual activity involving bodily functions of this kind should be treated very carefully when there are transmittable diseases in the mix. Make sure you, your partner and anyone else you choose to involve in your adventures is clean of diseases, or else do your research as to how to make a successful go at it when one partner is carrying a disease.

Shoe Fetish, Foot Fetish

You might think these two would be somehow connected – but tell that to a fetishist of one or the other, and you'd be saying fighting words! Shoe fetishists worship shoes in a sexual way, although often the act of a woman donning a shoe can also be intensely erotic. Foot fetishists adore only the bare foot; maybe an ankle or two. You've probably seen funny portrayals of these fetishes on Sex and the City, or in Something About Mary. Quentin Tarantino is said to have a foot fetish; watch his movies, and then you tell me.

Crush Fetish

This is a man masturbates as a woman wearing stockings and heels crushes bugs of varying size, the crunchier the better.

Furries
An episode of CSI: Las Vegas featured a furries convention! Furries dress up like stuffed animals (think team mascot types) and engage in rubbing against each other (frottage) and cuddle orgies. But, as Dan Savage would say, Furries Don't Fuck! They also don't speak, but instead grunt, mew, and make other sounds. They rarely reveal their human selves.

Octoporn
This is mostly portrayed in porn, but is becoming increasingly popular enough to warrant a mention. In octoporn, women are photographed or filmed with an octopus strewn over their bodies. I really don't know if they're live or not, and I'm afraid to ask.

Quicksand
Again, this is something that has come from porn portrayals and has gotten to the point where men build sand pits in their backyards for the purpose of masturbating while watching women get stuck in quicksand. No, I'm not sure how they get them out.

Breast Worship and Tit Fucking
Breast worship is where the man masturbates while burying his head in a woman's breasts. Tit fucking involves thrusting the penis between squeezed-together breasts.

Giantess Worship, Midget Worship
Yep, you guessed it: Tall girls and small girls.

BBW (Big Beautiful Women)

While this is a fetish, admirers of BBWs are more into relationships with these women than simply sex – although there certainly is a large fetish community of BBW worshippers. There are even BBW dances and socials that match up these big ladies with their fans.

Feeders

Feeders become sexually excited by feeding women. Unfortunately, this can take an incredibly dangerous turn as the fetish escalates to the point where the man wants the woman to become so large as to not be able to leave the house.

Sex Dolls, Real Dolls

You might think of a sex doll as some gag gift, a blow-up Sally that comes in a little box. But there are men who spend thousands of dollars on anatomically correct, eerily lifelike figures that they buy full wardrobes for, speak to, travel with and more.

Voyeurism

There are many different kinds of voyeurism. For example, you can watch your mate have sex with someone else from a hidden vantage point (with everyone's consent, of course). But "Peeping Toms" are also voyeurs, and can get arrested for it if caught!

Services

I personally know someone who, once a week, is paid $500 to allow a man to come into her house, clean it from top to bottom, masturbate in the bathroom, and then leave.

Stockings and Panties
Men who fetishize stockings either want them on the foot of a woman, or perfectly new out of the box. Panty worshippers want them worn and unwashed.

Asphyxiation
In asphyxiation play, you want your partner to cut off your air supply so that your orgasm is more intense. I can't begin to stress strongly enough how dangerous this is. Please, do not attempt it.

Infantilism
Men who have an infantilism fetish ARE NOT attracted to infants or are in any way pedophilic. Instead, their excitement is derived from being an infant themselves. They dress is diapers, cry and speak like babies, and particularly enjoy soiling themselves and having a woman clean them afterward.

Cling Film
Despite the description I'm about to describe, this is a man's fetish. A woman wraps a man entirely in plastic wrap – yes, like the kind you use for leftovers – leaving only enough for him to breathe. Then he stands or lies immobile and watches the woman masturbate. This is also called mummification fetish.

Caging
You might think this would be a part of female domination, but it's actually most common among gay men and men who put women in cages. While in the cage, the person behaves like an animal, is fed like an animal and

communicates like an animal. Within this fetish, there are people who will insist that it's only valid if one barks like a dog as opposed to meowing like a cat, and vice versa.

Fisting

I did not include this in anal play because it is in another category than those who are excited by anal play. Fisting can be either anal or vaginal, and it more the act of the fist being inserted than simply the penetrative aspect. For vaginal fisting, there is an added element of excitement once the entire fist is inside and the man opens his hand.

Women's Bodily Functions

While each of these are a separate and distinct fetish, I'm grouping them all together under one heading. These fetishes include menstruation fetish, pregnancy fetish, lactation fetish and douching or enema fetish.

Lingerie

Sure, you like to see your ladylove in a sexy teddy. But eventually, you want that bad boy to come off, right? Not so with lingerie fetishists. They enjoy lingerie, and women in lingerie, but purely to look at or touch while masturbating.

Vampire

This takes a biting fetish to another whole level – or rather, within the vampire fetish community, is considered an entirely different kettle of fish. Vampire fetishists of both sexes enjoy having teeth capped to be pointed, biting to draw blood, tasting blood and cutting to draw blood.

SAFETY is a major issue with this fetish, and everyone should test negative for disease before even contemplating this.

Piercing

The fact that this is a fetish does NOT mean that all people with piercings are wearing their heart on their sleeve, so to speak. There are some who eroticize the act of piercing, while others like to touch, fondle, kiss, lick or suck piercings.

Scent

While scents from perfume to fresh-baked cookies can warrant their own fetish, a scent fetish refers to the eroticism of one's body's natural scent. This can get pretty ripe, and simply unhygienic, so it's important to know the body's limits.

Pain

I really don't want to get into the extremes of pain-based fetishes, but I'll give you some examples – hot candle wax dripping, nipple pinching and clamping, whipping, knife play, medieval devices, excessive spanking or paddling, hair pulling, torture, and branding, to name a few.

• • •

I'm sure you've had your fill. Let's move on!

Chapter 10: Inviting Others to Play

Many kinds of sexual experimentation can lead to multiple-partner experiences in the bedroom. Assuming that you have a rock solid, trusting relationship, there is nothing to fear when inviting others into your sexual relationship.

However, guys, this doesn't necessarily mean simply a threesome with your lady and her gal pal – as much as lesbian sex is near and dear to your hearts. There are many combinations and kinds of group play that come under the heading of multiple partner games, and I cordially invite you not only to read about them here – but to be open to your partner's fantasies, too. Even if that means that, heaven forbid, you're in the same room with another naked man.

One of the most common issues that arise when either partner has a fantasy involving people outside of the relationship is that there might be some feelings of inadequacy. Am I not enough for him? Does she want to break up with me? Is he bored? Has she been cheating on me? What's wrong with just me?

These and more are all normal initial reactions to the idea of multiple partner experimentation.

This is the time to really bring out the heavy guns in terms of making sure she knows that this is something you want to explore together. Even if your fantasy involves you having sex with another person, it's crucial that you include her in the entire process and reach compromises whenever possible.

But this tactic is not for only your fantasies. In order to encourage your partner to talk about her own fantasies, put her at ease by saying that you understand this doesn't mean she doesn't love you and want to be with you. Sexual experimentation of any kind is just that – experimentation done by two loving people who are looking to explore the boundaries of their sexual feelings, desires and abilities. While it brings your relationship closer together, by no means is sexual experimentation to be seen as a comment on or reaction to the relationship you share.

Ready? O.K., let's do it!

Like some more extreme experimentation we've talked about, group play really shouldn't be the first thing you try right out of the gate. Role play and gender play can be a good warm-up, as can extended dirty talk involving group play scenarios, especially when combined with sex toys (i.e., your penis in one orifice and a dildo in another, with you describing your fantasy of a threesome with her and another male; or, eating her out while you penetrate her with a dildo and talking about a threesome with another female).

No matter how you get to that point, there are some important considerations when entering into group play:

- The person or people you choose for your adventure should be agreed on by both of you, with no coercion.

- Some couples choose to play with people they know; others wouldn't dream of it; still other couples prefer to hire a professional. This is entirely up to you, but again should be something that is decided upon mutually beforehand. You don't want to pop the question to a buddy and have her freak out because she hates him, or she springs on you that she found someone who's coming over in a bit, and you're not remotely attracted to him or her.

- There should be some discussion as to how one imagines the evening to go – will you be meeting up just for sex or will you be doing other activities (dinner, drinks, bowling?), what happens afterward (do you want to get the person out the door, or can they stick around?), whether or not you want it to happen in your home, theirs, a hotel room or some other location, etc. Even if you agree that it can happen spontaneously, you don't want to be trying to catch her eye or give her awkward signals that this is not what you had in mind.

- There should be a safe word you agree on with your partners, as well as a separate one for the two of you, so that if one of you gets creeped out or freaked out your partner will back you up.

- No matter what the combination, always be prepared with plenty of protection. Do not assume the other person will have it.

- If you've chosen to meet up with strangers, have a contact who will call you or you call them at a certain time to make sure you're both O.K. No, this is not a pussy move – this is smart planning. While it is extremely rare, there are those who take advantage of just your type of desire.

- Another thing to think about beforehand are your sexual parameters. What are you and are you not willing to do, and what is a deal-breaker for her? You don't want to get into a fight in the middle of a hot session because someone suggests something that one of you definitely doesn't want to do.

- Talk to your new partner(s) about their desires, goals for the session and what they will and won't do, too. Be as specific as possible without killing the mood!

Now that we've gotten that out of the way, I'd like to get into the particulars of the many kinds of multiple partner play with which you and your girl can experiment. Please note that no matter what kind of activity you choose that involves other people, trust me – there are entire communities devoted to it, both online and off. Do your research (always together!), and get acquainted with the people in these groups.

This can go a long way, by not only becoming familiar with the scene itself, but, you'll be much more comfortable if you arrive at a group event and already know people there, and what to expect.

You'll also learn how to integrate multiple-partner experimentation into your relationship from people who have done it, and can better tell you about it after they've learned of your particular dynamic. It's a comfort to know that this kind of experimentation is more common than you think among loving couples in committed, long-term relationships.

But, the best part about meeting people who are into multiple partner activities is that you and your mate will come to realize that they're not sexual predators, sex addicts or freaks of nature who spend all their time fucking. They're perfectly normal people, some with families, some with high-level jobs, some with not-so-high-level jobs, of every age, ethnicity and background.

You're sure to find someone you connect with, and you just might be surprised to discover how welcoming these communities are!

Threesomes

Whether it's FFM or MMF, threesomes can definitely bring some excitement to the bedroom. But it's also the most intimate, with the odd-partner-out really getting a sense of their partner having sex with another person. Make sure you are both psychologically and emotionally ready for the impact of that visual. No matter if it's been your fantasy for a while, try to get an image in your head of you, sitting or lying or standing there, while another person touches the love of your life. Ask your ladylove to do the same, and make sure you're in it to win.

Couple Swapping

When two couples get together, a variety of combinations can take place – so again, it's important all four of you have it worked out beforehand so no one gets bent out of shape – in a bad way.

- The four of you swap partners, either having sex in separate rooms, or all together in the same room. This can be done at the same time, or alternating, with the odd-partners-out watching one couple have sex at a time. Mutual masturbation can be a part of this as well.

  - You have sex with your own partner, as do they, while you're all in the same room.

  - You swap partners to make two same-sex couples.

  - You switch it up; anything goes.

Swinging

Swinging generally defines a group sex event in which multiple couples swap partners or engage in other sexual activity on a large (i.e., larger than simply two couples) scale. While two females getting it on in a swinger scene is accepted, each swingers' group has its own rules for male/male activity, so it's best to check ahead if this is what floats your boat.

Polyamory and Open Relationships
This is on a more extreme level – it's when one or both partners in a relationship have long-term or emotionally intimate relationships with others outside the base relationship. Not for the faint of heart, it is absolutely imperative that everyone involved is on the same page before entering into this type of relationship agreement.

Group Sex
While group sex is technically defined as any sex in which there are more than two participants, the thing that sets apart true group sexual activity from other types is that it is truly a group – there is very little or no splitting off into smaller numbers, and many times one person can be having sex with multiple partners at the same time, who are having sex with other people as well.

A "daisy chain" is the perfect example of this – it is literally a chain of people who are giving and receiving oral sex at the same time.

In group sex practices, there can be couples, singles, gay, straight, and bisexual in attendance – anything goes.

Cuckolding
Cuckolding, plainly put, is when a woman cheats on her man. However, there is an entire fetish surrounding this act, mostly connected with female-dominated relationships.

Your relationship has got to be solid as the Rock of Gibraltar for this to be an exciting, successful fetish.

The man can or cannot be present while the woman is having sex with another man (it's overwhelmingly heterosexual cuckolding with this fetish). If the man is not present, he might help her choose her clothes for her "date," or they might get together afterward so that she can tell him all about it in detail, either while having sex or in addition to withholding sex as part of the female domination aspect of their relationship.

If the man is present during the cuckolding, he may or may not be allowed to pleasure himself while watching his partner have sex with another man. Also, the cuckolding may or may not immediately be followed by sex between the couple.

Impregnation and Pregnancy Fetish

Impregnation fetish is just what it sounds like – you and your partner fantasizing during sex that you are impregnating her, or that you both just found out she is pregnant, or any combination of her, you and a fictional baby you're making or have made together.

There are two distinctly different camps of this fetish, the most popular by far being simply between one couple; however, I bring it up here because it can involve cuckolding or other kinds of multiple-partner sex.

When it is with only you and your partner, it can be as described above, and you can even go so far as to have your partner don a fake belly.

When it is a part of the cuckolding fetish, the fantasy involves the "other man" having impregnated her, and his sperm being stronger than yours, and several other kinds of (agreed-to) humiliation.

Interracial Fetish
Many couples combine role-playing, multiple-partner sex, cuckolding or an impregnation fetish with the fantasy of one or the other partner having sex with someone of a different race.

Homosexual Experimentation
Either one or the both of you can experiment with members of the same sex during almost any one of the above multiple-partner scenarios. This includes pre- and post-operative transsexuals, transvestites, drag queens and kinds and "chicks with dicks."

This does not mean you or your partner are gay.

Prostitute/Escort Fantasy
I'm including this at the end of this section not because it is so kinky or edgy, but because in many places it is just plain illegal, and you should be knowledgeable about the law in your area and the consequences for breaking it.

Having been thus far educated in the ways of experimental sex, you can probably guess that:

1. Your woman probably won't be into this idea right off the bat.

2. Role-playing, dirty talk, and mutual interest in advanced fetishes can open her up to inviting the paid trade into your relationship.

So, do your research, involve your lady, and discuss your options. A note here – if you have a prostitute fetish that involves street walkers, I strongly urge you to hire a high-end escort to play out this fetish with you and/or your partner, for your personal and physical safety as well as your health.

Conclusion

Well, here we are at the end of our time together. We've been through a lot!

If I may, I'd like to take a moment to summarize what we've learned in class today, kiddies.

No matter how tame or extreme your fetish might be, there are some hard and fast rules (oh, the puns!) that come with any kind of sexual experimentation.

First, everything I've described or recommended in this book is for long-term, monogamous couples. If that describes your relationship, then go for it!

If you're not sure, ALL of the following adjectives should describe your present relationship:

- Solid
- Committed
- Monogamous (at least before experimentation, depending on what you're thinking of doing)
- Long-term (married, engaged, living together or otherwise exclusive for a lengthy amount of time)
- Trusting

- Communicative
- Open-minded
- Loving
- Sexually active
- Fun, playful
- Emotionally intimate

All that notwithstanding, even the most equal, amazing relationships can have a bit of friction – and not the good kind – when it comes to sex and sexual experimentation.

I've said it a million times already, and I'll say it one last time: OPEN COMMUNICATION IS THE MOST ESSENTIAL REQUIREMENT for anything that happens in the bedroom. It doesn't matter if you're with a Late Bloomer, a Normal Girl, a Tantalizer or a Wild Child – you've got to keep those lines of communication open.

But, that doesn't mean that you'll be doing all the talking and convincing. Nothing else – not money, not the future, not wedding plans, nothing – is more of a two-way street than your sex life. You have to figure out a way not only to talk to her about your ideas, fantasies and fetishes, but to listen to her, too.

Listen for how she phrases her reactions to what you're saying. You know her well, so read her body language – is she tense, or wrapping her arms around herself, or perhaps leaving the room to do an errand in another during the conversation? These are all signs that she is not being receptive to what you're saying.

HOW TO GET HER TO...

If this is the case, then you need to let it rest for a while and try to find a new way to bring it up again at a later date. Maybe you were a bit judgmental? Did you bring it up at the wrong time? Perhaps your were a bit too excited, or you came across as being selfish? Rethink your strategy and try again.

Part of that strategy is knowing exactly what you are into, and knowing how to explain it. Remember, guys, we love you, and we want to please you – so show us that you care, too, and think about what you're saying and how you're saying it.

Take into account your woman's background. Was she chubby as a child, teen, or even since fairly recently? Is she overweight now, or has been complaining about her weight?

How about how she was brought up. Is her family deeply religious, or was she raised in a very strict home? Do you ever get the idea that she and her friends talk about sex and relationships, or does it seem like she's with a more closed off crowd?

And, of course, you must take her own sexual history into account – and not just with you. Has she had any trust problems with ex-boyfriends? Has she ever been the victim of any kind of abuse? Does she have any serious relationships under her belt? Was she assaulted, date raped or does she know someone close who was? Has she had an abortion? What's her take on feminism when it comes to sexual relationships?

CONCLUSION

Depending on the type of woman you are with, you should be able to gauge how slowly and carefully you should take any kind of sexual progression in your relationship. To repeat from an earlier chapter, just because I thought it was so awesome and true:

Here are some things to keep in mind:

- Always keep the focus on the two of you doing it together, as true partners in sex.

- No matter what your prior experience is, NEVER, UNDER ANY CIRCUMSTANCES, can you tell her about other girlfriends who've been into being dirty with you. Never. EVER. Lie, if you have to, within reason.

- Keep calm when you're talking about it, especially after she becomes more open to the idea. You don't want to act like a kid who just got a puppy.

- The same goes for including her in the conversation – keep her involved, and LISTEN to her. Don't just ask her a question so that she'll ask you back, and give you your chance to unload everything.

- Be open and understanding to what she's saying – no judgments, no laughing AT her, no being embarrassed. She might tell you things that she's ashamed of, or that she has been told are bad or weird. Reward her trust in you.

HOW TO GET HER TO...

No matter what your kink, those are basically the rules.

But, as always, I have more to say:

- Be physically safe. Don't put yourself in physical danger.

- Your health is your priority. Make sure anyone you involve in your sexcapades is disease-free. Always use protection, especially when involving other people.

- Practice good hygiene, especially for the messier stuff.

- Be mature. These are adult games you are playing in a further expression of your sexual side. Sexual experimentation should not be used to repair relationships or because you are bored.

- Be discreet. You are doing this because you love each other and want to bring your relationship even closer than it is already. This is not for bragging rights at the bar, or to be used to get other people in bed. You need to be in agreement on who gets to know how much of what you do behind closed doors, if anyone, or if ever.

- Be patient. You've purchased this book because you have been having a hard time getting your partner to open up sexually. I've given you much advice and many answers here, but none of it will happen overnight. You're going to have to take it slowly and make sure she is on the same page as you every step of the way.

- Learn to compromise. Depending on what it is you're interested in, you might have to come to terms with the fact that you may never get exactly what you desire in the bedroom.

This last point is an important one that I wanted to save for this conclusion.

If you follow the information I've given you, you will be able to get your partner to open up in the bedroom. However, there are certain things that even the most adventurous of us will never do – or, it might just be that your girl is just plain less sexually adventurous than you.

If, despite all of the hard work you've both done, you come to an impasse on your wildest sexual dream, it's time for you to review your options.

If her not agreeing to your fetish is a deal breaker, then break the deal. But you'd better be really, really sure.

You can stay in the relationship, but agree with your spouse that you will find someone – preferably a professional, to avoid sticky emotional ties – to indulge you.

You can satisfy your urges with porn films, photographs and literature that cater to your fetish.

You can compromise, which can entail several combinations. Either she does what you want to do in exchange for something – anything – she wants to do; or, if she is flatly against it, you can perhaps come to a lesser agreement – maybe she talks about it with you while you're having sex, or writes you letters about it, or whatever.

No matter what option you choose, it is your responsibility to involve her in the decision-making, and arrive at a solution together. While I have a great deal of respect for the pull of sexual desires, in no way do I, or anyone in the fetish community, condone going behind your faithful partner's back in search of sexual satisfaction.

It is my sincere hope that the information contained in this book, put into practice, brings you and your mate closer together than ever before. Exploring one's sexuality and sexual limits, can be a powerful force in a relationship dynamic. Once you bring your partner along on this journey of discovery, you might find that other aspects of your relationship are strengthened and you create a bond that lasts a lifetime filled with pleasure and love.

However, I'd like to include here something that I wrote in a previous chapter.

> *Sexual experimentation of any kind is just that – experimentation done by two loving people who are looking to explore the boundaries of their sexual feelings, desires and abilities.*

Conclusion

While it brings your relationship closer together, by no means is sexual experimentation to be seen as a comment on or reaction to the relationship you share.

This is a very important piece of information to keep in mind, and one that should be brought up repeatedly while discovering your sexual selves together.

So, go forth young man, and create your sexual future with your mate at your side!

Also from Secret Life Publishing:

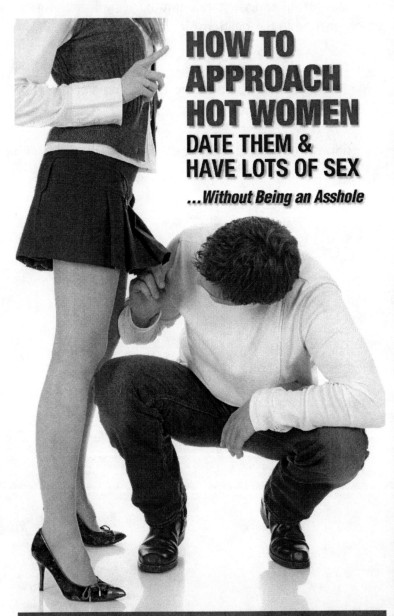

Palmer Strong

GUIDE TO EATING OUT

The Lick-by-Lick Guide to Mouthwatering and Orgasmic Oral Sex

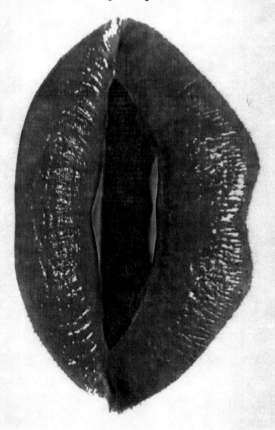

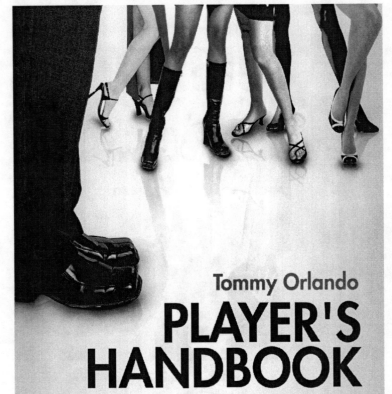

Tommy Orlando

PLAYER'S HANDBOOK

For Men Who Love Women & Sex
(and Want More of Both)

VOLUME 1
Pickup & Seduction Secrets

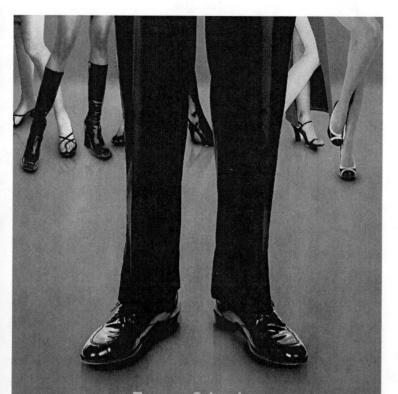

Tommy Orlando

PLAYER'S HANDBOOK

**For Men Who Love Women & Sex
(and Want More of Both)**

VOLUME 2
Advanced Pickup &
Seduction Secrets

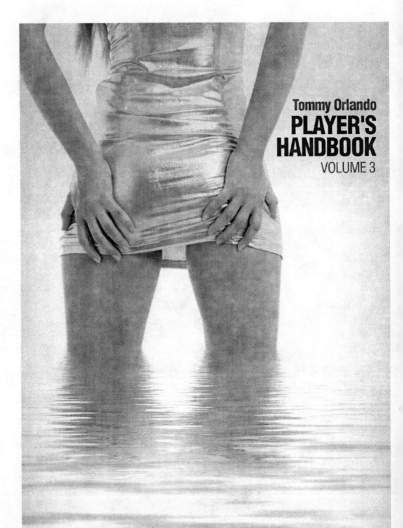

Tommy Orlando
PLAYER'S HANDBOOK
VOLUME 4

WHAT TO EAT
(AND HOW TO EAT IT)
A QUICK AND DIRTY GUIDE TO GIVING GREAT ORAL SEX

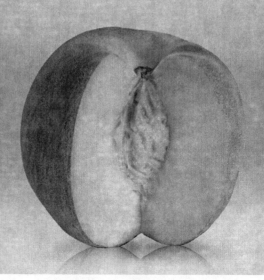

LaVergne, TN USA
27 January 2010

171350LV00001B/57/P